KT-463-274

Drug Safety
A Shared Responsibility

Drug Safety
A Shared Responsibility

Written by

International Drug Surveillance Department (IDSD)
Glaxo Group Research Ltd, Greenford,
Middlesex, UK

Foreword by
Michael D. Rawlins BSc MD FRCP (Lon) FRCP (Edin) FFPM
Professor of Clinical Pharmacology,
University of Newcastle upon Tyne, UK

CHURCHILL LIVINGSTONE

EDINBURGH LONDON MELBOURNE NEW YORK AND TOKYO 1991

CHURCHILL LIVINGSTONE
Medical Division of Longman Group UK Limited

Distributed in the United States of America by Churchill
Livingstone Inc., 650 Avenue of the Americas, New York,
N.Y. 10011, and by associated companies, branches and
representatives throughout the world.

© Glaxo Group Research Limited, 1991

All rights reserved; no part of this publication may be
reproduced, stored in a retrieval system, or transmitted in
any form or by any means, electronic, mechanical,
photocopying, recording or otherwise, without either the
prior written permission of the Publishers (Churchill
Livingstone, Robert Stevenson House, 1–3 Baxter's Place,
Leith Walk, Edinburgh EH1 3AF) or a licence permitting
restricted copying in the United Kingdom issued by the
Copyright Licensing Agency Ltd, 33–34 Alfred Place, London
WC1E 7DP.

First published 1991

ISBN 0 443 04655 7

British Library Cataloguing in Publication Data
A catalogue record for this book is available from the British
Library

Library of Congress Cataloging in Publication Data
available

Printed in Great Britain by Butler & Tanner Ltd, Frome and
London

Foreword

Drug safety is everyone's concern. Patients, pharmacists, prescribing doctors, regulatory authorities and pharmaceutical companies all have an interest in ensuring that medicines combine the
maximum efficacy with the minimum of toxicity. Absolute safety –
zero toxicity – is, however, unattainable and even the most innocu-
ous drugs may very occasionally be hazardous. We must all therefore be alert to the possibility that medicines may sometimes cause
harm.

Drug Safety—A Shared Responsibility is written by the members
of the Drug Safety Department of a major international pharmaceutical company. It will be reassuring to members of the public
and the health care professions that the industry takes such a
rigorous view of its responsibilities. The book, itself, will be of
special value to pharmacists and physicians with responsibilities
for drug safety whether they work in hospitals or the community,
regulatory authorities or the pharmaceutical industry. I also hope
that undergraduate students of medicine and pharmacy will take
advantage of its contents: the future of drug safety is largely in
their hands.

1991   M.D.R.

Preface

The importance of safety surveillance of medicines has increased greatly in recent years. Worldwide, more and more people are becoming involved in the reporting of adverse reactions and the role of general practitioners and pharmacists is becoming increasingly important all the time.

This book was produced to fulfil a need for a basic introductory text to the subject of adverse reaction reporting. It is aimed particularly at pharmacists, medical students and general practitioners. Some areas are only covered briefly, but we hope that interested readers will follow up with further reading. Whilst all the authors work for Glaxo Group Research, we have tried to write a general text book using examples from our own experience where useful to the reader. The book was a team effort and many members of the International Drug Surveillance Department, who were not chapter authors, made significant contributions.

We hope as a result of this book that there will be an increase in awareness and reporting of adverse drug reactions. To do the best for the patient we all depend on each other.

Greenford, Middlesex, 1991   IDSD

Acknowledgements

We would like to thank all those within Glaxo who made it possible for us to turn our idea for this book into a reality. We are particularly indebted to Dr Goran Ando for his interest and encouragement, and to Allen & Hanburys for financial assistance.

The authors and managing editor greatly appreciate the indirect contribution of all members of the International Drug Surveillance Department, who not only showed constant interest and enthusiasm for the project but also bore with great good humour, continual office interruptions and information overload on the topic of 'The Book'! Special thanks are due to Simon Brooks, David Solomon and Liz Swain for their editorial input, and to Rosemary Beach for preparation of the index. We are extremely grateful to our ever-willing secretaries Julie Dunn, Ganchana Emptage, Julie Friend, Debbie Knight and Alison Ryan for preparation of original manuscripts and to Maria Turner who typed the final draft.

An expression of gratitude is also made to Judith Maconochie for her review of chapter 2 and also to Martin Redman for commenting on chapter 6.

Finally a word of thanks to the staff at Churchill Livingstone who have been enthusiastic and encouraging at all the right moments.

Greenford, Middlesex, 1991   IDSD

Contributors

Pamela A. Adams BSc Cert.Ed. (Managing Editor)
Principal Clinical Research Scientist,
International Drug Surveillance Department (IDSD),
Glaxo Group Research (GGR), Greenford, UK

Niall W. Balfour BSc MSc
Clinical Research Scientist, IDSD

Elliot G. Brown MB ChB MRCGP BMedSci DipPharmMed MFPM
Senior Research Physician, and Head of Medical Group, IDSD;
Formerly Senior Medical Officer, Medicines Control Agency;
Head of Medical Affairs, Sanofi (UK) Ltd, UK

Win Castle MD FFPM MFCM MB BS MIS
Director, IDSD; Former Head of Product Safety ICI
Pharmaceuticals; Reader in Epidemiology, University of
Birmingham, Zimbabwe, Africa

John Freeman BSc DipClinSci.
Senior Clinical Research Scientist, IDSD

Cathy J. Griffiths BSc MRPharmS
Clinical Research Scientist, IDSD; Former Hospital Pharmacist,
UK

Peter J. K. Gruer MSc (Epidemiology) MBChB MRCP (UK)
Research Physician, IDSD

Amanda J. Jukes BSc MRPharmS
Principal Clinical Research Scientist, IDSD;
Former Hospital Pharmacist, UK

Neelam Patel BSc
Clinical Research Scientist, IDSD

Sue M. Roden BSc MSc MRPharmS
Head of Drug Review Group, IDSD;
Former Hospital Drug Information Pharmacist, UK

M. D. B. Stephens MD FFPM MRCGP DObstRCOG DMJ
DipPharmMed RCP
Consultant and Former Head of Safety Evaluation, IDSD

John C. C. Talbot B.Pharm MSc PhD MRPharmS
Head of Spontaneous Reports Group, IDSD

Lesley J. West PhD DipInfSci
Systems Advisor, IDSD; Former Senior Scientific
Officer ADR section (now Pharmacovigilance), MCA;
Adverse Event Co-ordinator, Bayer UK Ltd, UK

Lewit A. Worrell BSc ASc
Clinical Research Scientist, IDSD

Contents

1. **An introduction to drug safety surveillance** 1

   Benefit–risk ratio
   The unpredictable nature of side-effects
   Recognizing side-effects
   Adverse events versus adverse reactions
   Classification of adverse drug reactions (ADRs)
   Data sheets
   Specification of incidence rates
   Other sources of side-effect data
   The patient's perspective
   The role of the health care professional
   The role of the drug industry
   The role of the regulatory authorities
   Sue M. Roden

2. **They test new drugs don't they?** 13

   Toxicological evaluation
   First use in man – phase I studies
   Phase II and III studies – the real testing ground?
   The role of investigators in safety monitoring
   Detection of adverse drug reactions in clinical trials
   John Freeman

3. **Post-marketing surveillance** 27

   Further clinical trials
   Beyond clinical trials: epidemiological studies
   Cohort studies
   Case-control studies
   Problems in pharmacoepidemiology
   Post-marketing surveillance (PMS) studies

Prescription event monitoring (PEM)
Record linkage and PMS
Individual methods of drug surveillance
Peter J. K. Gruer

4. **Spontaneous reporting** 37

The role of spontaneous reporting
Limitations of spontaneous reporting
What can and cannot be done with spontaneous reports
Comparing spontaneous reports with different drugs
Factors influencing spontaneous reporting
Source of spontaneous reports
Obligations of pharmaceutical companies
Company databases
John C. C. Talbot

5. **Has the patient suffered an ADR? – assessment of drug causality** 47

Mechanism of ADRs
Detection of ADRs
Differential diagnosis
Methods of causality assessment
M. D. B. Stephens

6. **The interface between the medical profession and the pharmaceutical industry** 57

Reasons for reporting suspected ADRs to manufacturers
Barriers to reporting ADRs directly to manufacturers
Safeguards and reassurances
Expectations of reporters and the industry
Controversies – Direct reporting by non-medically
qualified persons
– Payment for adverse reaction reporting
– The actions taken by pharmaceutical
companies in response to reports of
adverse reactions
Elliot G. Brown

7. **An overview of the role of industry**   67

Why does industry monitor the safety of its drugs?
Sources of data for the industry
The company databases
Approaches to data review
Decision making
Identifying subgroups at particular risk
Estimating the frequency of the adverse reaction
Communication
Win Castle

8. **How to report suspected adverse drug reactions
(ADRs)**   77

The origin of ADR reporting
The Yellow Card scheme
The reporting of ADRs to the pharmaceutical industry
What the pharmaceutical company does with the data
Niall W. Balfour

9. **Medicines Control Agency (MCA) and other regulatory
authorities**   89

Introduction to the role of the regulatory authorities
Structure and function of the MCA
Life cycle of a drug licence in the UK regulatory authority
The CSM and Pharmacovigilance
Pharmaceutical companies and UK regulations
What the CSM do with the data
Standardization of the role of worldwide regulatory authorities
Lesley J. West

10. **The people working in the field – careers in drug safety
monitoring**   99

What does industry offer?
Working in drug surveillance
Drug surveillance at Glaxo
Regulatory authorities
The Health Service
Further career options
Cathy J. Griffiths, Amanda J. Jukes

11. Information sources 109

Published literature
Searching the literature
Searching information sources
John C. C. Talbot, Lesley J. West

Glossary 117

Neelam Patel, Lewit A. Worrell

Index 123

1. An introduction to drug safety surveillance

Sue M. Roden

The safety of medicines is of considerable importance to everyone. Modern medicines are expected to be efficacious, but will there be unwanted side-effects? What are they likely to be, and is it possible that they could be worse than the disease being treated? These questions are equally important to the manufacturer who has invested many years of research and development in producing the drug and to the reviewers at the regulatory authority who, having examined the tomes of information on these activities in the company's product licence application, has agreed, for the present time at least, to grant it a licence for the marketplace. However, it is not so easy as it might initially seem to provide answers to these questions and, for this reason, the science of drug safety surveillance has evolved.

In the first part of this chapter the basic principles of benefit–risk ratios, the recognition and classification of side-effects and data sheet statements will be examined. Because these factors are under continuous observation throughout the entire life span of a drug, their accurate characterization depends firmly on everyone who takes, dispenses, prescribes, manufactures or licenses the drug. That is, we all have a shared responsibility for monitoring drug safety.

BENEFIT–RISK RATIO

With the advent of more effective and novel drugs we need to be able to balance their therapeutic efficacy (benefit) with their liability to cause side-effects (risk). Not only should it be possible to evaluate the benefit–risk ratio for the potential patient population as a whole, but also the clinician needs to be able to assess the risk and benefit of each drug he or she prescribes for his or her individual patients. Clearly, the use of an effective drug with serious

1

side-effects is more acceptable in a patient with a potentially fatal disease, than the use of a similarly toxic but effective drug in a patient with a self-limiting disease. But do we know what the side-effects of a drug are? How are they detected so that the risks can be measured?

THE UNPREDICTABLE NATURE OF SIDE-EFFECTS

In some undergraduate pharmacology courses it is implied that each drug has a well-defined group of therapeutic and adverse effects. If this were the case, then testing drugs in a few thousand patients before marketing would be sufficient to identify all of the potential problems and no further post-marketing safety sur- veillance would be required. However, this simple approach does not allow for individual patient variation.

Drug action is unpredictable because of differences in drug hand-ling between patients; these differences may be in absorption, distribution, metabolism and excretion from the body. In addition, concurrent disease states may contribute to the manifestation of certain adverse drug reactions. For example, there is an increase in ampicillin rashes in patients with glandular fever, and vincristine-induced peripheral neuropathy is more prevalent in patients with Hodgkin's disease than in other cancer patients. We are therefore interested to determine both the effect of the drug on defined patient populations and the effect of these populations on the drug.

THE LIMITATIONS OF CLINICAL TRIALS IN DETECTING SIDE-EFFECTS

As will be discussed in chapter 2, at the time of approval most drugs have been studied in only a few thousand patients in carefully controlled clinical trials which are primarily designed to evaluate the efficacy of the new compound, often in comparison with its 'gold standard' (e.g. a new antidepressant versus amitriptyline). In these studies there are many exclusion criteria so that the drug may not be administered to elderly patients, neonates, pregnant women, or those with impaired renal, hepatic or cardiovascular function. However, these are the high-risk populations to whom drugs are frequently prescribed in general clinical practice.

Clinical trials will characterize common side-effects but not those occurring more rarely (an incidence of less than 1 in 250 patients treated). In addition, the drug's longterm safety is unknown as only a few hundred of the few thousand patients will have received it for longer than 1 year. Consider the example of the practolol-induced oculomucocutaneous syndrome which was not detected until after approximately one million patient-years of exposure, at least 4 years after approval was granted.

RECOGNIZING SIDE-EFFECTS

The practolol example also illustrates other problems in identifying side-effects of drugs during both pre- and post-marketing surveillance. Firstly, there had been no evidence in chronic animal toxicity testing that immunological abnormalities associated with ocular, mucous membrane, peritoneal or cutaneous changes may occur in man. Secondly, the syndrome is not known to occur with other β-blocking agents and thirdly, the unusual and unexpected nature of the effects on the skin, eyes and peritoneum demanded astute clinical observations to establish the relationship with practolol. This emphasizes that the clinician needs to be aware that new symptoms and signs occurring while patients are receiving drug therapy may be side-effects, and not simply separate additional diseases which in turn require additional drug therapy.

How then can side-effects of drugs be recognized? Unfortunately, there is no easy answer since many present as naturally occurring diseases. For example, is the pulmonary embolus occurring in a hospitalized patient receiving a new antibiotic due to the drug or would it have occurred anyway in this bed-ridden patient? For this reason it is common practice among doctors and scientists working in drug safety surveillance to collect all adverse events (AEs) occurring whilst a patient is receiving a new drug, so that they may be both counted and assessed for a drug-induced causality at a later date.

ADVERSE EVENTS VERSUS ADVERSE REACTIONS

So far, the terms side-effects and adverse effects have been used to describe the unwanted effects or toxicity associated with a drug but they do not specifically discriminate between concomitant AEs and true adverse drug reactions (ADRs). For this purpose an AE is defined as 'a particular untoward happening experienced by a patient, undesirable either generally or in the context of his disease' (Finney 1965). In contrast, an ADR is defined as 'any response to a drug that is noxious and unintended and that occurs at doses used in man for prophylaxis, diagnosis, or therapy, excluding failure to accomplish the intended purpose' (Karch & Lasagna 1975). The term adverse reaction implies a causal relationship with the drug, and an investigator who considers that, on balance, the pulmonary embolus mentioned in the earlier example was due to the patient's underlying pathology, may not report its occurrence. However, it may be that the new antibiotic increases the incidence of pulmonary emboli and this would only be evident if AEs are collected in comparator studies.

Classification of ADRs

ADRs have been divided into two basic classes, type A and type B (Rawlins & Thompson 1977).

Type A (augmented) reactions are pharmacologically predictable from the known activity of the drug (e.g. dry mouth associated with the anticholinergic action of tricylic antidepressants); they are common, dose related, generally not clinically serious and are associated with relatively low mortality. Because they are both common and expected they are usually identified before marketing.

Conversely, type B (bizarre) reactions are unpredictable, rare, not dose related, usually clinically serious with a relatively high mortality and are due to a hypersensitivity or an idiosyncratic mechanism (e.g. agranulocytosis associated with beta-lactam therapy).

At the time of marketing it is probable that only the more common and pharmacologically predictable ADRs will be known. After marketing, and for the entire duration of a drug's life span, continued safety surveillance is required to identify the rare, more serious ADRs and to study the safety profile in selected populations of patients (e.g. children or those with renal failure). This can be done either with formal post-marketing surveillance studies, as described in chapter 3, using epidemiological techniques (also described in ch. 3), or with spontaneous reporting systems as outlined in chapter 4. The end point of all these activities is to identify new adverse reactions and attempt to quantify the risk to the patient.

As ADRs are detected, or as new specific patient populations are identified as being at increased risk of developing side-effects, this information is added to the product's data sheet, which is intended to enable the doctor to prescribe it safely.

DATA SHEETS

In the UK, data sheets are prepared by the pharmaceutical manufacturer to comply with the requirements of the UK Medicines
Act 1968 and follow the requirements stipulated by the Medicines
(Data Sheet) Regulations 1972. Although the style may vary
between companies, each data sheet conforms to the standard
format shown in Table 1.1; they are updated regularly as it is in
everyone's interest that the information is as accurate as possible.
The appropriate data sheet is enclosed with each drug package for
use by the medical profession, and a copy is collated in the annual
Association of the British Pharmaceutical Industry (ABPI) Data
Sheet Compendium which is issued to all doctors and to pharmacies
by the ABPI. When major changes are made individual companies

Table 1.1 The format of the data sheet

1. Presentation	–	informs the prescriber of the physical appearance of the formulation and how much drug it contains.
2. Uses	–	gives the indication for use (e.g. may specify which organisms an antibiotic is effective against).
3. Dosage and administration	–	includes the dose recommendation for adults and children, the need for reduced doses in certain circumstances (e.g. renal failure) and, if necessary, details concerning the reconstitution of the product and the method and site of administration.
4. Contraindications, warnings, etc.	–	statements regarding safety data. Includes contraindications, precautions, use in pregnancy, drug interactions, side-effects and the management of overdose.
5. Pharmaceutical precautions	–	details on special storage conditions.
6. Legal category	–	indicates whether the drug is a prescription only medicine (POM) or can be bought from pharmacies (P).
7. Package quantities	–	gives the number of unit doses per pack.
8. Further information	–	intended for any other information relevant to the prescriber.
9. Product licence number	–	the number allocated by the regulatory authority when the drug is approved for marketing.

undertake to distribute updated copies either by post or via their representatives.

Data sheets are required by law in many other countries, although their format and content is not necessarily as described. In the UK it is only necessary to include the main side-effects and adverse reactions likely to be associated with a drug, and for that reason many manufacturers do not include every AE that has ever been reported with their product regardless of a causal association. However, it is sometimes thought that this may leave them vulnerable to litigation and there is an increasing tendency towards the philosophy of the USA where all possible side-effects are included. Clearly, many factors must be considered when deciding what safety information needs to be included in a data sheet.

Specification of incidence rates

Some regulatory authorities require that an estimate of the incidence of each adverse reaction listed be included in the data sheet. In some cases incidence figures such as 1 in 1000 are quoted but other regulators prefer terms such as frequent, occasional, and rare, and define the ranges for which these adjectives apply. Unfortunately, there is no current agreement upon these definitions which therefore vary in meaning from country to country.

A statement on the incidence of side-effects may initially appear to be valuable information on which to assess the benefit–risk ratio of various drugs. However, there are practical difficulties with obtaining this information especially from spontaneous AE reporting systems where neither numerator nor denominator are accurately known. Although these reports are invaluable for generating signals, considerable under-reporting occurs which varies between drugs, with severity, seriousness, type and uniqueness of reaction, the length of time the drug has been on the market, associated publicity and many other factors. Estimation of the total number of patients exposed is possible, but probably inaccurate, since it is necessary to rely on either worldwide sales data, rather than number of prescriptions, or selected data provided by agencies such as Intercontinental Medical Statistics (IMS) which may not be representative of the true experience.

Other sources of side-effect data

Apart from the product data sheet, other readily available reference sources on side-effects include the *British National Formulary* (BNF), *Martindale – The Extra Pharmacopoeia* and the *Monthly Index of Medical Specialities* (MIMS). More specialized references include *Meyler's Side-Effects of Drugs*, (annuals and editions), *Textbook of Adverse Drug Reactions* by Davies and *Iatrogenic Disease* by D'Arcy & Griffin. Further details of reference sources are discussed in chapter 11.

OUR SHARED RESPONSIBILITY FOR SAFETY SURVEILLANCE

Thus far this chapter has introduced the reader to the fundamental concepts of drug safety surveillance with its inherent difficulties. It is indeed a fascinating and stimulating area for research! It has been seen that new drug-related side-effects may emerge several years after drugs have been licensed for marketing and that there is a need for continual vigilance for their detection. But whose responsibility is this?

In the remainder of the chapter this question will be approached from the perspectives of the patient, the health care professionals (i.e. doctors, pharmacists and nurses), the pharmaceutical industry and the regulatory authorities, and we shall examine what contribution each can make.

The patient's perspective

In the last 20 years public debate about risks, benefits and drug safety has intensified and patient action groups are being formed to seek litigation against prescribing doctors and the pharmaceutical industry for drug-associated injuries. One of the common complaints is that patients are not given sufficient information about the potential side-effects of the medicines which they are prescribed. There may be many reasons for this including the severely restricted time available during consultation, the doctor's concern that the patient not be worried unduly, or the belief that if the patient is informed about the side-effects of a drug he or she will develop them all!

Most pharmaceutical companies in the UK are now providing patient guidance leaflets (PGLs) to be dispensed with their medicines. These are similar to product data sheets but written in nonmedical English, and, at present, are not a legal requirement. They contain common side-effects (which should be described in terms that the patient can understand), give details on the action to be taken if any of them are experienced and recommend that further information can be obtained from the patient's doctor or pharmacist. But what about those side-effects not mentioned in the patient leaflet?

Theoretically, the patient is in a key position to contribute to drug safety by communicating with his or her doctor or pharmacist. In practice this may not occur because the patient may not connect the event with the drug therapy, may fear being labelled as neurotic or may simply forget. Patients prescribed short courses of therapy may stop treatment prematurely because of side-effects but not consider it necessary to notify the doctor. Others may assume that all drugs have side-effects so they must tolerate them and not complain.

In summary, it must be recognized that new adverse reactions may go unnoticed unless patients are encouraged to report unusual events to their doctor or pharmacist.

The role of the health care professional

Once the patient has brought an event to the attention of a health care professional further obstacles must be overcome before it is reported to the pharmaceutical industry or to the regulatory authority. As mentioned earlier, the doctor may fail to recognize that the event is an adverse reaction, instead considering it to be a naturally occurring abnormality, or part of the disease, a complication thereof or a new disease state. Other factors inhibiting doctors reporting reactions are discussed in detail in chapter 6.

Although only those AE reports received from doctors or dentists are accepted by the UK regulatory authority, pharmacists, nurses and possibly other health care providers also have a contributory role in safety surveillance both in the community and in hospitals. Patients may confide their adverse experiences to the pharmacist during drug counselling sessions, or to the nurse who has greater contact with the patient than does the doctor. In addition, both hospital- and community-based pharmacists may be alerted to possible adverse reactions by noting concurrent drug therapy which may have been prescribed to treat a reaction, or by observation of the patient specifically for adverse reactions. Hospital-based clinical pharmacists, who see the complete medication chart, visit the wards and attend clinical ward rounds, and nurses caring for the patient, are in an ideal position to discuss the possibility that a new drug has caused an adverse reaction, and to persuade the busy houseman to report it, if appropriate.

The pharmaceutical industry receives a number of reports directly from pharmacists, of which some are extremely well documented. However, as the UK regulatory authorities only accept reports from doctors, it is important that pharmacists state when the suspected reaction has been medically confirmed so that it is evident that it needs to be reported by the company to the Committee on Safety of Medicines (CSM). Often clinicians may simply ask pharmacists for side-effect information to rule out the drug from the differential diagnosis.

The role of the drug industry

The pharmaceutical industry has two major roles in drug safety surveillance. First, it must promote the collection and investigation of information relating to adverse reactions for the purpose of advising on drug safety. Second, it must fulfil its obligation to the regulatory authorities by reporting individual AEs on an expedited basis and/or periodically, according to the regulations in each country in which a drug is licensed for clinical trial or marketing.

It is clearly in the company's interest to be the first to know that there is a potential problem with its drug so that appropriate decisions can be made. Very rarely it may be necessary to withdraw the product from the market either permanently, or temporarily until further information becomes available. Sometimes warnings are issued to prescribers to limit the use of the drug in specific populations, e.g. women of child-bearing age. This information may be disseminated in the form of 'Dear Doctor' letters. More often amendments are made to the data sheet and prescribers are sent updated copies. Similarly, if problems are identified during pre-marketing clinical trials the company will notify every doctor individually who is entering patients into the drug studies and also update their investigator's brochure appropriately to fulfil their obligation to both parties, i.e. doctors and patients.

But what data do companies use to identify potential safety issues? As described in subsequent chapters the drug safety surveillance departments of most large pharmaceutical companies have access to extensive computerized databases into which AEs from all volunteer, pre- and post-marketing trials are entered together with spontaneous AE reports from worldwide sources and reports from the literature. These data are reviewed regularly to identify as yet unexpected ADRs ('signal generation'), and to test hypotheses. If there appears to be a 'signal' then the appropriate case reports are examined in detail to assess the causal relationship with the drug. Once a judgement has been made that the potential side-effect is valid then the necessary measures are instituted and the appropriate interested parties worldwide, including the regulatory authorities, are notified.

The role of the regulatory authorities

Like the pharmaceutical industry, the regulators review all safety data for potential new problems; a full account of their activities is given in chapter 9. Sometimes they will be alerted to signals before the manufacturer because they receive reports directly from the medical profession. When this occurs they will discuss the situation with the company who then review their own data and make modifications to their data sheet as considered appropriate by both parties.

Occasionally manufacturers are requested to add 'class statements' to data sheets, e.g '... has been reported with cephalosporins' even if there have been no reports for their particular product. This is usually as a result of a regulatory review of a specific group of drugs from different manufacturers. It is argued that this undermines the value of identifying the specific ADR profile of each individual drug and also is not helpful to the clinician who may use the data sheet to decide which particular drug of a class to prescribe.

Apart from scientific evidence, the regulatory authorities are subject to political and media pressures to take action. This has sometimes been inappropriate and led to the premature withdrawal of innocent drugs from the market. On balance however, the prime concern of the authorities, like that of the industry, must be public health.

CONCLUSION

This introductory chapter was intended to set the scene for the rest of the book which examines in more detail drug safety monitoring, the methods employed and the reliance placed upon clinicians, pharmacists, patients and regulatory authorities. So, please read on and decide in your own mind where your personal contribution lies.

REFERENCES

Finney D J 1965 The design and logic of a monitor of drug use. Journal of Chronic Disease 18: 77–98
Karch F E, Lasagna L 1975 Adverse drug reactions. Journal of the American Medical Association 234 (12): 1236–1241
Rawlins M D, Thompson J W 1977 Pathogenesis of adverse drug reactions. In: Davis DM (ed) Textbook of adverse drug reactions. Oxford University Press, Oxford, p44

2. They test new drugs don't they?

John Freeman

INTRODUCTION

The introduction of any new medicine to the market will have been preceded by many years of development by the pharmaceutical company. For many involved in the prescribing, dispensing or administration of this new medicine, the exact nature of its pre-marketing development is probably unclear. Prescribers, dispensers and patients alike place great trust in the work that has brought that medicine to the market place, but what, precisely, is involved?

The first thing that can be said is that the development of a new medicine is not a quick and easy process; it is not simply a question of synthesizing the active constituent, tableting the compound, administering the drug to a few animals and human volunteers and then arranging for distribution to High Street chemists. The actual process from initially synthesizing the drug, establishing that it possesses the appropriate pharmacological action, and then ascertaining that it is safe and efficacious in man, may take 10 years or more to achieve. The development of new medicinal products is becoming increasingly complex and now demands an amalgamation of medicine, statistics, pharmacology, toxicology and computer data processing. The level of expertise required within pharmaceutical companies today bears little resemblance to that of even 10 years ago; the majority of professionals now entering the pharmaceutical industry find themselves poorly equipped and have to set about getting to grips with the new 'machinery' of pharmaceutical development.

Why should pharmaceutical development be such a complex state of affairs, and what are its principal features?

All drug regulatory agencies throughout the world now demand that any drug that is to reach the market should be subjected to rigorous evaluation to determine whether it is both safe and efficacious. The emphasis is primarily upon safe usage, although, amidst a market place full of similarly acting medicines, proof of efficacy is invariably required. Many drug regulatory agencies now look for a complete benefit–risk assessment, and balance the positive aspects of the drug against the known adverse effects within a pharmaceutical 'see-saw'. The initial emphasis on the determination of safety is easy to appreciate; in the early days of pharmaceutical legislation, the impetus for setting down requirements had much to do with the thalidomide disaster and practolol side-effects (see ch. 1).

The other big change during this period concerns the difference in the nature of drug development required by individual national regulatory agencies. Many pharmaceutical companies now indulge in a single, universal development programme, which has been made possible by an element of harmonization between regulatory agencies.

Five stages of development can be identified that provide the safety data essential in allowing the passage of drugs from the laboratory to the market. Following a pharmaceutical company's decision to develop fully a newly identified chemical entity, the first of the five stages is a study of the drug's animal toxicology. The clinical programme, split into four phases (I-IV), will commence during the latter stages of the toxicological evaluation.

TOXICOLOGICAL EVALUATION

Animal toxicity studies are the subject of regulations determined by the drug regulatory agencies. This series of studies, conducted over the course of several years, aims to reject toxic compounds and identify the drug's target organ of toxicity. Toxicity studies vary depending upon the intended use of the drug. In general, an increase in the duration of exposure in humans demands an increase in animal toxicity studies. There are five general types of toxicity study:

1. Acute, single dose
2. Subacute, subchronic, medium term
3. Fertility, teratology and reproduction
4. Carcinogenicity
5. Special studies (e.g. possible effects on neurological systems)

Perhaps the most widely discussed acute study is the LD_{50} – the

Table 2.1 Requirements for multiple dose studies

Duration of studies within animals	Human exposure permitted
14 days	1–3 doses
28 days	10 days
3 months	1 month
6 months	Indefinite

single dose of the drug which produces a fatal outcome in 50% of the animals treated within a 7-day period. A 'ball park' figure is sometimes required in two or more species. The LD_{50} test, provides, where used, a gross indication of the overall toxicity of the drug and is provided more for historical reasons than for its scientific value.

Multiple dose studies follow on from acute, single dose studies and are required before humans are exposed to the new drug. The requirements for multiple dose studies are determined by the intended duration of human dosage as shown in Table 2.1. These studies must be performed on two separate species, one of which should be a non-rodent. (If indefinite use is envisaged within man, carcinogenicity studies need to be performed). Three dose levels are selected, the lowest of which is comparable to the expected human dose, whilst the highest either should produce some evidence of toxicity or should be very much greater than human exposure levels.

Further studies for potential teratogenicity and effects on fertility and reproduction are almost universally required by the drug regulatory agencies. Teratological evaluation is usually required before the drug may be administered to women of child-bearing age. This evaluation is performed on the rat, mouse and rabbit and, at various stages of gestation, females are sacrificed and fetuses assessed. Fertility studies are carried out on both males and females, and involve dosing 60 and 14 days pre-coitus, respectively. Further studies permit completion of the reproductive cycle and the study of both parents and offspring.

Carcinogenicity studies are required only when the drug is intended for chronic (>12 months) use or, alternatively, if the drug may be used for repeated courses over long periods. These studies may also be required if the drug's structure suggests a carcinogenic potential or if mutagenicity studies (bacterial muta-genicity/Ames test) reveal any specific concerns.

Special studies to evaluate the effects of the drug on specific body systems tend to be performed only if particularly indicated by the results of earlier toxicological evaluation. These studies are often of effects on sensory systems.

By the time the battery of animal toxicity studies has been carried out, the drug's target organ of toxicity should have been defined. Additionally, the maximum tolerated non-toxic dose will have been established, and dose levels causing mortality in the long term may have been demonstrated.

Extrapolation of animal toxicity to man is very difficult. Thus, toxicity findings are only acceptable if there is a substantial safety margin in dose findings of organ-specific toxicity. The general consensus of opinion is that the responses of laboratory animals to drugs may differ from the responses of man. The causes of variation may be attributed to differences in metabolism (both qualitative and quantitative), distribution and pharmacodynamics. This is an area of intense interest, and important papers identifying and characterizing interspecies variation were written as long ago as the early 1960s (Oliverio et al 1963, Brodie & Read 1967).

As a result of the toxicological evaluation the most toxic agents will have been eliminated; however the final experimental model has to be man. Clinical development is split into four phases (I–IV). The early trials in man are executed with great care and initially use only very low doses – these are the first of the phase I studies.

FIRST USE IN MAN – PHASE I STUDIES

In contrast to other clinical studies which are performed before a new drug reaches the market, phase I studies are designed primarily to evaluate safety. Phase I consists of initial testing of a study drug in humans, usually in healthy volunteers but occasionally in patients.

Of all the clinical studies performed, phase I studies are the most rigorously monitored, with the subjects being confined to a highly specialized facility for at least 24 hours following a single admin-istration of the new drug. Most major pharmaceutical companies have an in-house facility for performing phase I work, although independent units have been established in association with many teaching hospitals and offer phase I evaluation on a contract basis.

Aims of phase I

The principal aim of a phase I study is to permit progression to phase II. It therefore aims to assess tolerability within a dosage range which will include and exceed that likely to be given to patients at a later stage. From this early evaluation should emerge an indication of the nature and severity of pharmacologically predictable and dose-dependent adverse drug reactions (ADRs), the so-called type A ADRs. The dose at which these types of effects occur should be characterized, and some indication may be provided as to whether the reaction is transient and may subside with continued administration. As something may be learnt of the drug's pharmacokinetics during phase I, it may be possible to relate drug body fluid levels to the emergence of type A reactions, which are dose-dependent.

There is no absolute progression from phase I to phase II. Phase II studies invariably commence midway through any phase I development and phase I studies may still be performed once a drug is marketed.

Methods used during phase I studies

It is not difficult to picture the scene within a phase I facility during the first ever administration of a new drug to man. A volunteer (invariably a healthy young adult male) receives a low, single dose of the new drug amidst a team of white-coated staff, surrounded by equipment common to that located in most intensive care units. The observations that are made of subjects during phase I evaluation include:

- 12 lead ECG determinations
- Continuous cardiac monitoring and Holter analysis
- Blood pressure and pulse
- Blood sampling for drug assay if appropriate and for haematological/biochemical evaluation
- Continuous subject observation
- Regular clinical examination
- Specific observations related to the drug's therapeutic class e.g. psychometric and EEG evaluation

The very first use of a new drug in man may be surrounded by an element of nervous anticipation and excitement, but as soon as the dosing and observation of the first group of subjects is complete it is time to move on to the next dose level. The single dosage is increased in a pre-defined manner either until the estimated therapeutic dosage has been exceeded, or until the maximum tolerated dose is obtained. The selection of the dosages to be employed at this stage derives entirely from the animal toxicology data, with fractions of doses (mg/kg) associated with the first toxic pharmacological effect being employed. Normally 8 volunteers are studied at each dose level – typically 5 receiving active drug and 3 receiving placebo (Rogers & Spector 1986).

Only upon completion of single dose studies can multiple dose studies begin. Usually, the new drug is administered in much the same way as in subsequent patient treatment. Dosing periods vary from 7–28 days. The dosing interval is typically one half-life, providing this is known, otherwise once-daily administration is selected. The observation of subjects is as intense within multiple dose studies as it was in single dose studies, although it is unlikely that (despite being institutionalized) subjects would be confined to bed. Kinetic data are determined principally during multiple dose studies. The doses employed are ideally those which achieve steady state blood levels below those which produced toxicity in the single dose studies. Groups of 8–12 subjects are studied with placebo control, and there are typically 6 such studies in total. Approximately 48–60 subjects in total will therefore have been studied.

Messages from phase I evaluation

As far as assessing the safety profile of new drugs is concerned, phase I studies are very limited. The most that can realistically be expected from this phase is the characterization of common type A ADRs. In view of the limited number of subjects studied, only the most common events will tend to be observed. The incidence of such events during phase I tends to be very different from that determined during subsequent clinical trials because of the extensive monitoring of subjects.

If the drug undergoing evaluation belongs to a known class of compounds, it may be appropriate to extend dosing to levels sufficient to induce less severe type A reactions. The information obtained from this exercise may, by comparison with existing drugs, be predictive of the likelihood of patients experiencing the same event. The other sort of information which may emerge concerns the likelihood of a particular type A reaction to subside with continued treatment; this is not uncommon for some type A reactions but is clearly dependent on severity.

Information obtained during toxicological evaluation may be placed under scrutiny during phase I and it may even be appropriate to design specific protocol observations on the basis of such considerations.

Serious toxicity is rare during this early stage of development. To the best of the author's knowledge, no fatalities associated with immediate anaphylaxis have ever been reported. The more bizarre and unpredictable type B ADRs tend not to be encountered during phase I as they are so rare, and are usually only detected after marketing.

Safety data from phase I studies have considerable limitations, as only healthy subjects are being studied and they do not exert any of the modifying influences which may be due to disease states. There is little scope within healthy subject studies for there to be variation in the body's absorption, distribution, metabolism or excretion of drugs. This may not be so in a patient environment where, despite inbuilt safety checks, patients with hepatic or renal impairment may occasionally enter studies. It is really only in this wider forum that more extensive detail of the drug's safety profile emerges. Although, having stated that, it will be clear from the later discussion that even when the completion of phase III is achieved, the full safety profile still remains to be elucidated.

PHASE II AND III STUDIES – THE REAL TESTING GROUND?

At some point during the latter stages of phase I, studies in selected populations of patients commence. These are patients for whom the drug will eventually be indicated. These first studies in patients are referred to as phase II; they tend to be relatively small and may even be regarded as pilot studies for the more extensive clinical evaluation that is phase III. Phase II aims to define an effective dose of the new drug in closely monitored and controlled conditions. The information provided by phase II is utilized in the design of phase III studies which are large scale and of longer duration.

Phase II differs from phase I in that the latter was designed primarily to evaluate safety – the main aim of phase II is to establish efficacy in a patient population and to permit the choice of an appropriate dose. Thus, safety assessments tend to be secondary to those of efficacy during this phase. The aims of phase III evaluation are shared equally between safety and efficacy. Phase III observations are the principal source of data for the product's data sheet. Phase II and III combined will usually have studied 1000–2000 patients; of these a large proportion will have been treated in a clinical setting comparable to that which will be employed after the drug has been marketed.

Study design utilized during these phases will vary according to the stage of development, therapeutic area under consideration and whether there are relevant comparator products on the market. As many as 40–50 separate studies may be performed, although the largest proportion of the 1000–2000 patients will have been studied in no more than three or four longer-term studies. The execution of studies is closely controlled by drug regulatory agencies and all protocols require separate approval.

The detection of ADRs during phase II and III

The number of studies performed and the number of patients likely to be included in them were described earlier. In what is a closely monitored clinical setting, with what would appear to be large numbers of patients, phase II and III development might be expected to answer any safety question that may arise. Unfortunately this is not the case – one only has to consider some of the more recent drug safety problems to appreciate the limitations of pre-marketing clinical trials in detecting ADRs.

It is generally considered that clinical trials in this phase of development are capable of identifying type A ADRs that affect 1 in 250 patients studied. This is the level of information that will then appear within a new drug's data sheet. If, however, the incidence of some of the less common but more serious type B ADRs is considered, the inherent limitations of this stage of a drug's development are brought home. Type B ADRs, in contrast to type A, are neither pharmacologically predictable nor dose related. Type B reactions tend to be rare, are usually serious and have either a hypersensitivity or an idiosyncratic mechanism. The estimated incidences of examples of such events are given in Table 2.2.

Given the indicated incidence of known ADRs, it is also possible to estimate the number of patients required to be exposed to the drug during clinical trials for these ADRs to have been detected

Table 2.2 Estimated incidence of some examples of type B reactions

Drug	Adverse drug reaction	Incidence
Chloramphenicol	Aplastic anaemia	1/6000
Halothane	Jaundice	1/10 000
Oral contraceptives	Deep vein thrombosis	1/10 000
	Myocardial infarction	1/10 000

(assuming, of course, that the event in question may be causally attributed to the drug only and not to some other cause). Table 2.3 provides an indication of the number of patients required to detect 1, 2 and 3 ADRs for five different expected incidences.

It must be emphasized that Table 2.3 assumes that the event does not occur other than because of drug-induced causes i.e. there is no background incidence. If we look back at Table 2.2, in which the estimated incidences of some of the known ADRs were listed, it is quite clear that the likelihood of detecting these reactions during studies of 1000–2000 patients was remote. A further assumption made here is that the reaction was recognized at all!

Against this background, one could question the validity of expending vast amounts of effort, time and finance on investigating safety during phase II and III development. There is a place for safety monitoring at this stage; it rests largely with identifying firstly those safety statements which should subsequently appear on the first version of the new product's data sheet (under the side-effects and warnings section) and secondly those safety hypotheses which may subsequently be tested after marketing.

Table 2.3 Numbers of patients required to be treated to detect adverse reactions

Expected incidence of adverse reaction	Number of patients required to be treated for occurrence of following numbers of adverse reactions:		
	1	2	3
1 in 100	300	480	650
1 in 200	600	900	1300
1 in 1000	3000	4800	6500
1 in 2000	6000	9600	13 000
1 in 10 000	30 000	48 000	65 000

(From Lewis 1981)

The role of investigators within phase II and III safety monitoring

Clinical trials during phases II and III of a drug's development, particularly phase II, tend to be performed within hospital-based departments specializing in particular areas of medicine. It is not usual for studies to be performed by general practitioners although some may be set up (in appropriate circumstances) during the latter stages of phase III. Pharmaceutical companies frequently find themselves 'competing' for centres and patients with other companies, and one option now adopted by most large companies is the initiation of international, multicentre clinical trials. A protocol describing all procedural elements of the study will be available, together with a structured means of documentation – the clinical record form.

Safety is assessed on a prospective basis by obtaining baseline, pre-treatment data and then continuing to collect data during periods of treatment with the study drugs. The two types of data described below are obtained and a variety of methods employed:

1. Clinical signs and symptoms are recorded throughout the study as a result of scheduled clinical examinations and patient consultations. Patients may be allowed to volunteer details of any health problems that have occurred, may be prompted to provide this information, or may be required to complete a checklist which is then discussed with the investigator.
2. Laboratory assessments are also made at defined periods during the conduct of trials. The most common being examination of urinary, haematological and blood-biochemistry parameters together with ECG measurements. Other clinical measurements may be made where specifically indicated.

It is imperative to the successful evaluation of safety within trials that all details requested within clinical record forms are properly completed by investigators when recording safety experience.

The diagnosis of ADRs is extremely complex. It has already been indicated that the likelihood of encountering anything other than a common (< 1:250 incidence) ADR is slim, let alone actually attributing drug causality to it once identified. For this reason, the assessment of ADRs in clinical trials tends to be statistical and uses large pools of patient data within the context of an overview. This approach raises probably the single greatest cause of difficulty and misunderstanding between clinical investigators and pharmaceutical companies. This is because the industry now collects safety data involving not only ADRs, but also adverse events.

Protocols defining safety procedures generally instruct investigators to record all medical events within the safety sections of clinical record forms, regardless of the investigator's own ideas of drug causality. This procedure permits the recording of both 'background noise' and true ADRs in a manner which allows future analysis of pooled data to statistically 'dissect out' possible ADRs, using direct comparison between drug-treated and placebo- or comparator-treated groups of patients. This approach is perfectly valid but its main downfall is the very damaging effect of investigators failing to document patient experience as they believe that the drug could in no way cause a particular event. This is particularly troublesome in situations where the very disease which is being studied commonly breaks through. Perhaps the best example involves studies of anti-asthmatic drugs where symptoms of asthma are regularly reported during the study period. As troublesome as it may seem, there is a real need for investigators to document all such occurrences so that each patient's experience may be married up to that of others and comparisons between treatment groups made.

The scene back 'in-house' during phases II and III

An outsider considering pharmaceutical development may be forgiven for imagining that once clinical trials are underway the industry staff involved take a 3 month holiday whilst waiting for the data to arrive back from clinical investigation – this is far from the truth!

This period is often the busiest for pharmaceutical personnel and this is no exception for those involved in safety surveillance. Many companies now have departments whose sole responsibility is the safety surveillance of both drugs undergoing development and those which are marketed (see ch. 10).

Clinical trial protocols will invariably require investigators to make two types of safety report during the conduct of clinical trials – one for immediate notification to the company and one for collection by company staff upon completion of the study. Pharmaceutical companies are obliged to provide safety information to drug regulatory agencies worldwide following receipt of certain 'immediate notification' reports from investigations. Companies are permitted only a short period of time (which may be as little as 3 days) to submit a regulatory report following receipt of a report from an investigator. To achieve this on a worldwide basis companies tend to utilize extensive databases. Staff on the receiving end of 'immediate notification' reports from investigators have a responsibility, therefore, to investigate the adverse event report in order to clarify its nature and then to convey that information to appropriate drug regulatory agencies. This is the reason that the pharmaceutical personnel involved in this aspect of drug safety monitoring may often be perceived as having more than just a passing interest in obtaining further information within the shortest timeframe possible!

The further investigation of adverse event reports by the drug industry is something that often perplexes the investigators who may feel that a particular patient's recent medical event was entirely due to non-drug causes. The pharmaceutical industry has a considerable obligation to investigate fully adverse event reports, not only to permit the submission of appropriate reports to drug regulatory agencies but also to be certain that the adverse event bore no causal relationship to the drug.

In situations where it is suggested, or even certain, that a drug in development has caused an adverse event (at which point it is renamed an ADR), the pharmaceutical company has certain obligations. Firstly, the drug regulatory agencies need to be informed as discussed previously. Secondly the investigators themselves need to be notified. All drugs in development are the subject of an extensive document which is provided to all who are concerned with its clinical development. This document, known as the clinical investigator's brochure, carries details of the drug's clinical safety. Important, serious ADRs which have been identified are documented together with an indication of the less serious but more common suspected reactions. In addition to obligations concerned with notifying others of drug safety reports, the pharmaceutical company continually monitors the nature and number of adverse event reports that it receives for drugs within phase II and III development. This continual surveillance of new drugs aims to characterize the expected reactions and alert all concerned with the drug's development to serious, unexpected reactions. It is this latter aspect of drug safety surveillance which sometimes results in the abandonment of a drug's clinical development.

At the end of phase III development, perhaps 5 years after the first administration to man, a considerable amount of safety data will have been amassed. This invariably amounts to in excess of 2000 patients' experiences, many of whom may have been taking the drug on a chronic basis (dependent upon indicated use) for up to 12 months. The amount of safety data generated can be staggering – particularly if the disease state is associated with a high incidence of 'background noise'. This data has to be incorporated within an appropriately structured analysis which will form part of the drug's product licence application. The main purpose of this analysis is to highlight the ADRs which will form part of the drug's data sheet. Additionally, this analysis represents the most extensive review possible of the drug's safety prior to marketing. By structuring the analysis correctly, it is not only possible to determine the reactions to be included within the data sheet but also to comment on their characteristics and incidence. The analysis may also be structured to examine the effects of patient variables upon ADRs e.g. age, sex, race and concurrent medication. This latter aspect may permit the inclusion of information within either the 'warnings' or 'contraindications' sections of product data sheets. This analysis is often the basis for a number of hypotheses concerned with safety, which may then be investigated in studies after marketing and also monitored from adverse reaction reports made by physicians who have prescribed the drug.

AND FINALLY ...

The clinical development of new drugs is an expensive and lengthy process. The pharmaceutical industry is putting increasing effort into new drug development and is continually attempting to perform this process in an increasingly efficient and effective manner. The monitoring of drug safety during this period is, without doubt, of the utmost importance and is number one in the list of priorities. It is clear from the previous discussion that the responsibility for ensuring that safety monitoring is performed correctly rests with both the pharmaceutical company and clinical investigator alike – it is truly a shared responsibility. It has to be appreciated that for many reasons beyond the control of the pharmaceutical company, the drug regulatory agencies or the clinical investigators, the clinical development period is not the final testing ground as far as safety is concerned.

Essentially, pre-marketing evaluation forms just one small part of the drug's safety checklist. It is during the later stages, after the drug has been marketed and perhaps further larger studies performed, that more of the drug safety 'jigsaw' is completed. Data obtained during pre-marketing clinical development may only be effectively utilized in the light of experience obtained after market-ing. The pre-marketing data may contain one or two reports which were not regarded as being of importance until perhaps a further half a dozen are encountered following prescribed usage. In this respect, the data that formed the basis of the drug's product licence application may become very important as a source of reference information when dealing with subsequent safety experience.

The final test of the drug's safety starts when the first pre-scription for that drug is written and continues throughout the lifetime of the drug. Whether the observance of safety falls within one specific post-marketing study or with the observations made spontaneously by a prescribing physician, the absolute need for diligence and awareness of the importance of continued sur-veillance cannot be overstated. The procedures that form the basis of a new drug's safety surveillance after reaching the market are described in the next few chapters – large, formal, safety sur-veillance schemes will be described and a detailed review of pre-scriber/spontaneous reporting of adverse reaction reporting will be made. It will be clear that in common with the pre-marketing safety surveillance, that performed after marketing is also a shared responsibility.

REFERENCES

Brodie B B, Reid W D 1967 Some pharmacological consequences of species variation in rates of metabolism. Federal Proceedings 26: 1062–1070
Lewis J A 1981 Post-marketing surveillance: how many patients? Trends in Pharmaceutical Sciences 2 (4): 93–94.
Oliverio V T, Adamson R H, Henderson E S, Davidson J D 1963 The distribution, excretion and metabolism of methyl-glyoxal-bisguanylhydrazone-^{14}C. Journal of Pharmacology and Experimental Therapeutics 141: 149–156
Rogers H J, Spector R G 1986 Handbook of clinical drug research. Blackwell Scientific Publications, London

3. Post-marketing surveillance

Peter J. K. Gruer

Whilst the systems of spontaneous reporting (described in ch. 4) form the mainstay of safety monitoring for drugs that have passed from development into the market place, they are by no means the only methods employed; a variety of other techniques are used by regulators, academics, companies and independent bodies to continue monitoring and studying the adverse reaction profile of marketed drugs.

FURTHER CLINICAL TRIALS

The manufacturer's programme of clinical trials does not end when their new drug is granted a marketing licence. Usually an extensive programme of post-marketing phase IV studies is organized which involves a wider range of clinicians, centres and, indeed, countries than the pre-marketing studies. Phase IV studies are designed to test the safety and efficacy of the drug in common clinical practice and give individual physicians the opportunity to compare the new drug with their own standard therapies. Whilst these trials add usefully to the overall clinical experience with the new drug, they share the same constraints of numbers as pre-marketing trials and are therefore unlikely to lead to the identification of previously undetected problems.

Often the manufacturer will continue to conduct a number of additional phase II and III trials (see ch. 2) to assess the use of the new drug in indications and patient groups (e.g. paediatric) not included in the initial licence application. By thus exposing groups of patients with different risk-factor profiles, these studies may detect side-effects that were not seen, or were very uncommon, in the original pre-marketing programme.

Once the new drug is available on prescription, clinicians themselves may initiate trials with the new drug in patients with problems unique to their own speciality (e.g. nephrology, hepatology) and who may be more at risk of developing problems secondary to drug therapy.

Occasionally the company, or individual clinicians, will discern that in addition to a therapeutic role, a drug may have a use in primary or secondary prophylaxis. In any prevention study only a proportion of the 'at risk' group, whether treated or not, will develop the outcome (disease) of interest. As a result, prophylaxis studies tend to be considerably larger than therapeutic trials, and may identify previously unrecognized side-effects. However, before exposing essentially healthy individuals to longterm drug therapy, investigators must be confident the trial drug is safe. Prophylaxis studies therefore tend to involve older, well tried drugs which have well described adverse drug reaction (ADR) profiles.

Prophylactic studies have been most common in cardiovascular diseases, notable examples being the Coronary Drug Project (conjugated oestrogens, clofibrate and niacin) and the WHO clofibrate trial, reviewed in Bulpitt's *Randomised Controlled Clinical Trials* (1983)

BEYOND CLINICAL TRIALS: EPIDEMIOLOGICAL STUDIES

For a drug that proves commercially successful, the number of patients involved in the clinical trial programme, however large, will be small in comparison with the numbers of patients treated during the drug's marketed life. Where a drug has been proven to have a significant level of efficacy, and there is no evidence to suggest a significant safety problem, continuing to restrict its use to the patients of physicians engaged as clinical trialists, and indeed to leave the decision of which of those patients will benefit to the lottery of randomization, may no longer be ethically justified. The further study of a drug's safety must therefore rely on other methods of investigation. Since the mid 1960s the foremost of these methods have been systems of spontaneous reporting (see ch. 4). Increasingly, however, the methodologies of epidemiology are being applied to the study of drug safety. Epidemiological studies break down into two major groups – cohort studies and case-control studies.

Cohort studies

In cohort studies a group of individuals exposed to the drug are identified and followed up over a period of time to assess the rate of occurrence of ADRs. In most cohort studies of drug safety, a group of individuals prescribed the drug will be followed up and compared with another group not taking the drug (who act as a control), allowing the incidence of adverse events (AEs) in the two groups to be compared. It can easily be seen that this set up closely parallels the structure of clinical trials. The critical difference between cohort studies and clinical trials is that in the latter, patients are allocated to the study or control groups by randomization, whilst in the former, patients have already been prescribed the drug (or not) prior to being followed up.

Like clinical trials, cohort studies are best used to study one drug at a time but they can be used to study many outcomes simultaneously. They are therefore ideally suited to the monitoring of drug safety where many different AEs may arise in association with a single drug, and where the outcomes of interest cannot be defined in advance. Cohort studies allow the incidence of AEs to be measured, and have a structure similar to clinical trials and therefore their results are easily understood and accepted by professionals used to handling clinical trial data.

A major disadvantage of longterm cohort studies is that many subjects may be lost to follow-up. This reduces the power of the study to identify rare ADRs, by effectively reducing the numbers in the study, and may affect the validity of the results.

Cohort studies are very expensive; they inevitably involve a large number of patients and, for drugs taken chronically (to provide useful data), must continue for several months or even years. Whilst ideal for monitoring a wide range of possible side-effects, cohort studies are a very inefficient method for studying specific rare suspected adverse reactions. Obviously to study an AE occurring in 1:10 000 patients receiving the drug, on average, for every one patient suffering that event, 9999 patients receiving the drug but who never suffer the event must also be followed up (as well as 10 000 controls). Such investigations may be better carried out as a case-control study.

In clinical trials, patients are allocated the drugs to be studied. In cohort studies patients taking the drug and controls have to be identified from the general patient population; identification of these patients is a major stumbling block. In the UK the

Prescription Pricing Authority (PPA) co-operate with several agencies to identify patient cohorts. Other groups identify patient groups by writing to GPs and enlisting their help. Modern computer prescribing and record-keeping systems are now beginning to offer useful, quick alternatives.

Case-control studies

In case-control studies a group of patients with a particular disease (or ADR) are compared with a group who do not have the disease, and their histories of previous exposure to a 'risk factor' i.e. drugs or factors are compared. Case-control studies can thus best investigate one outcome (e.g. ADR) but can study the association with several exposures (e.g. drugs).

In drug safety work case-control studies have no role in monitoring, but can be invaluable in investigating specific drug-AE association hypotheses generated by cohort monitoring studies or by spontaneous reporting.

Earlier in this chapter we have seen that to study a rare suspected ADR many thousands of patients would need to be followed up using cohort study methods. By studying only individuals suffering the event (whether due to the drug or not) as well as one to four controls per case, a case-control study could investigate the same problem using tens of subjects, instead of the tens of thousands required in the cohort study.

The great advantage of case-control studies is their relatively small size, low cost and speed compared with cohort studies.

However, if not carried out rigorously case-control studies can be prone to biases from which cohort studies tend to be relatively free. This, plus their 'back to front' logic, tends to make them less readily accepted by professionals used to clinical trials. Although case-control studies can be used to establish an association between a drug and a suspected ADR, they do not allow the incidence of the effect to be measured. Well conducted case-control studies, however, can provide valuable insight into suspected ADR problems and are probably at present greatly under-used in drug safety work.

Case-control studies depend on the identification of patients who have suffered the disease or AE of interest. If fatal these may be identified from death certificates. For non-fatal cases computerized records in hospital and general practice, again, are beginning to offer useful sources. For certain conditions e.g. cancers, disease registries exist, and pressure is increasing for registers of other rare diseases e.g. blood dyscrasias, toxic hepatitis etc., to be set up to facilitate their study.

Problems in pharmacoepidemiology

Randomization of treatments in clinical trials ensures that the two groups are, on average, equivalent except for the drug they are receiving. Any differences between the two groups in AE incidences can therefore be assumed to result from the difference in treatments. In cohort studies it is most unlikely that the two groups are the same, and differences in AE rates are as likely to result from intrinsic differences between the patient groups as from their different drug exposure. False associations between AEs and drug usage can similarly arise in case-control studies.

Differences between groups can be reduced by 'matching' subjects with controls who are similar in important factors, such as age, sex, disease and disease severity. However, it is only possible to match for a few factors in any one study and important differences are likely to remain.

Differences between groups can be controlled-for to some extent during data analysis, using techniques of stratification and modelling. However, these techniques can only control for factors that have been accurately recorded for each patient. Recording such factors greatly adds to the expense and complexity of the study, and the subsequent analyses make the results much less 'transparent' to the reader who thus has to take results 'on trust'.

Patients taking a particular drug prescribed for a particular condition or disease may differ from those not taking the drug in factors associated with the disease for which they are being treated. A major source of false associations between a drug and an AE is this difference in the health status of subjects and controls. Overcoming this 'confounding' of treatment and disease is one of the major problems in carrying out drug safety epidemiology.

The need to overcome such problems when using epidemiological techniques to study drug safety has led to the birth of the discipline of pharmacoepidemiology. Already there are a number of books devoted to the subject and a number of universities, most notably McGill in Canada, now run courses in the subject. A number of societies, e.g. the International Society for Pharmacoepidemiology (ISPE), arrange meetings in the UK and elsewhere.

POST-MARKETING SURVEILLANCE (PMS) STUDIES

In recent years, it has become increasingly common for companies to set up what are known as PMS studies. PMS studies are cohort studies set up to monitor the safety of a drug in the immediate post-marketing period.

Pharmaceutical companies wishing to carry out PMS studies often enrol the services of one of a number of companies specializing in their design and operation.

As a rule, these companies ask a panel of GPs to send the follow-up details of the first 10 or so patients for whom they prescribed the new drug. The GPs may also be asked to send similar details on control patients taking a specified comparator drug. Usually these studies follow cohorts of around 10 000 patients, although this will vary from drug to drug depending, for example, on the 'size' of the indication.

In the past GPs were often given a significant fee for completing the follow-up medical report forms, leaving these studies open to the criticism that they might encourage doctors to prescribe the new drug for patients in whom they might not otherwise have used it. This criticism led to these studies being referred to by some as 'seeding studies'.

In an attempt to avoid abuse of these important studies the Association of the British Pharmaceutical Industry (ABPI), the Committee on Safety of Medicines (CSM), the British Medical Association (BMA) and the Royal College of General Practitioners (RCGP) have drawn up guidelines to which all company-sponsored post-marketing surveillance cohort studies should adhere. These guidelines are now published at the front of all ABPI Data Sheet Compendia. Perhaps the two most important 'rules' are: firstly that patients must be included in the study only after the decision to prescribe the drug has been made and not vice-versa and, secondly, that GPs are given fees proportionate to the work involved in completing the reports (agreed with the BMA) and not of a level which could be seen as inducements to prescribe the new drug.

To provide any useful information PMS studies must be large. The cost of ad hoc cohort studies of drug safety are therefore considerable, company sponsored studies involving 10 000 patients using a commercial investigator may cost in the region of £1 000 000. As a result, PMS studies of individual drugs by non-commercial groups are rare; independent sponsoring agencies with limited budgets, no doubt quite properly, believe that such studies involving individual drugs are the responsibility of manufacturers.

Independent studies are more important in studying the effects of classes of drugs where the market is shared by a number of individual products – a number of important independent studies have been carried out looking at the longterm safety of oral contraceptives (Kay & Hannaford 1988; Vessey et al 1989) and others have been proposed to study hormone replacement therapy (HRT) in peri- and post-menopausal women.

With financial assistance from the manufacturer, a group of eminent academics carried out a large PMS study of the H2–antagonist cimetidine in Glasgow, Oxford, Portsmouth and Nottingham (Colin-Jones et al 1982 & 1987). Patients filling a prescription for cimetidine (written by GPs participating in the study), were identified from local pharmacists' listings or from copies from the PPA. For each patient an age- and sex-matched control was recruited from the list of the patient's GP. About 15 months after a patient and control pair were identified the practice was visited again and their notes examined for all hospital referrals, deaths and adverse reactions noted by the GP. The study recruited almost 10 000 patients and 10 000 controls, and was reported in a number of publications. This study highlighted a number of problems encountered in PMS: the size and the amount of data collected are considerable; coding of the multiplicity of diseases, procedures, symptoms etc., had to use systems designed for other purposes and meant that great care had to be taken in retrieving information; the time taken between conception of the study in 1977 and the first publication in 1982, 5 years later, emphasized that PMS cannot provide instant results; perhaps most markedly it highlighted the problems of confounding between drug and disease.

Controls were matched for GP, age and sex, but not for peptic ulcer disease. As a result there were many differences between the cimetidine and control groups in the incidence of diseases such as ischaemic heart disease, lung disease, lung cancer and cirrhosis of the liver – which were due to the smoking and drinking habits of people with peptic ulcer disease – rather than any effect of the drug.

Prescription event monitoring (PEM)

PEM is a system of intensive surveillance of newly marketed drugs, run by the Drug Surveillance Research Unit (DSRU) in Southampton. The DSRU is managed by the Drug Surveillance Research Trust, an independent registered charity which is supported by 'no strings attached' grants from pharmaceutical companies and from the Department of Health. PEM, which was developed by Professor Bill Inman (who for several years managed the Yellow Card spontaneous reporting scheme at the CSM), is designed to supplement the Yellow Card scheme by providing more intensive monitoring during the early period of a drug's marketed life. The scheme takes advantage of the drug prescription system administered by the UK National Health Service. Every National Health prescription written by a GP in England is sent to the PPA. This allows remuneration of dispensing pharmacists, and provides information on the quantity and cost of drugs prescribed by GPs to the Department of Health and local Family Practitioner Committees (FPCs).

For selected newly licensed drugs the PPA, by arrangement, sends the DSRU a copy of each of the first 10 000 or so prescriptions (the number varies from study to study). The DSRU then sends a questionnaire (or 'green form') to the prescribing doctor requesting information on any health events suffered by the patient whilst on, or following treatment with, the drug in question. An event is defined as 'any new diagnosis, any reason for referral to a consultant or admission to hospital, any unexpected deterioration (or improvement) in a concurrent illness, any suspect drug reaction, or any other complaint which was considered of sufficient importance to enter in the patient's notes'. PEM has advantages over the Yellow Card Black Triangle system, firstly because it allows determination of the incidence of adverse reactions by providing a denominator, and secondly, in recording all AEs it can identify ADRs which may not be recognized for what they are by individual physicians, and which therefore may not be reported by Yellow Card. By actively seeking data from GPs the PEM system also enjoys a higher response rate than the 'passive' Yellow Card system. (For details of various aspects of the Yellow Card scheme refer, to chs 4, 8 and 9.)

Unlike company-sponsored PMS studies, as previously described, PEM studies do not require GPs to identify patients prescribed the new drug, and do not pay GPs fees for completing the report forms. This, together with the fact that studies are not commissioned by the manufacturer, means that PEM is free from the criticism directed at other PMS studies that they can be used to alter prescribing habits.

Record linkage and PMS

The use of computers is becoming increasingly common for the storage of medical records, drug prescription and practice management, both in hospital and general practice. This computerization of medical practice, by facilitating the linkage of prescription data with medical record data, offers a valuable resource for the study of drug safety.

In the UK, some companies who supply computers and software to general practices have arranged to receive automatically anonymous details of all prescriptions, diagnoses, complaints, hospital referrals etc., recorded by many client GPs.

These companies can thus now offer pharmaceutical companies an alternative to the paper-based methodologies previously employed in PMS. Computer-based PMS studies can be carried out, using routinely recorded data, without GPs being aware which drugs or patients are being studied. Studies using these systems could therefore avoid the criticism that they alter doctors' prescribing habits.

As the record-linked systems routinely capture and store prescription and event data, they not only provide facilities for prospective cohort studies, but also allow for rapid retrospective or case-control analyses in response to specific problems; since the data is collected prospectively the studies are not prone to some of the biases that can plague genuinely retrospective studies.

In Scotland, a system called MEMO, based in the University of Dundee, uses individual patients' unique community health numbers (which are not used in England and Wales) to link data from Scottish Hospital Morbidity Returns with prescriptions provided by the PPA. This group hopes to establish links with GP computer networks to capture, automatically, both prescriptions and GP-record events. They also hope to extend their population beyond that of the Tayside Region to which the system is confined at present. If they succeed in these aims they may then also be in a position to seek contracts for company sponsored studies.

INDIVIDUAL METHODS OF DRUG SURVEILLANCE

Beginning in the 1960s in Boston, Massachusetts, the Boston Collaborative Drug Safety Programme (BCDSP) intensively monitored 50 000 consecutive hospital admissions for drugs prescribed, ADRs, hospital discharges etc. The database resulting from this mammoth undertaking has been extensively used to study a variety of drug and ADR associations. Monitoring activities were discontinued some time ago, but the database remains available for studying older drugs.

In the United States, medical care is paid for by a variety of private health plans, health cooperatives and veterans' associations as well as the Medicaid system. The databases of a number of these organizations are regularly used to study drug safety.

In the Saskatchewan province of Canada each of the 1 000 000 population has a unique eight–digit number. This number can be used to link prescription data with physician and psychiatric service records, and cancer and vital statistics.

These databases do not routinely monitor drug safety, but can provide data for the investigation of specific drug and ADR hypotheses. Each database has its own strengths and weaknesses and these are widely reviewed and referenced by Stephens (1988).

CONCLUSION

In summary, after a drug is marketed its safety continues to be assessed in continuing clinical trials, using epidemiological techniques, and, most importantly perhaps, as described in the following chapter, by systems of spontaneous reporting.

REFERENCES

Bulpitt C J 1983 Randomised controlled clinical trials. Martinus Nijhoff, The Hague
Colin-Jones D G, Langman M J S, Lawson D H, Vessey M P 1982 Cimetidine and gastric cancer preliminary report from post-marketing surveillance study. British Medical Journal 285: 1311–1313
Colin-Jones D G, Langman M J S, Lawson D H, Vessey M P 1987 Review: post-marketing surveillance of the safety of cimetidine – the problems of data interpretation. Alimentary Pharmacology and Therapeutics 1 (3): 167–177
Kay C R, Hannaford P C 1988 Breast cancer and the pill – A further report from the Royal College of General Practitioners oral contraception study. British Journal of Cancer 58: 675–680
Stephens M D B 1988 Post marketing surveillance (PMS) In: Stephens M D B The Detection of new adverse drug reactions. 2nd edn. The Macmillan Press, Basingstoke 143–200
Vessey M P, McPherson K, Villard-Mackintosh L, Yeates D 1989 Oral contraceptive and breast cancer: latest findings in a large cohort study. British Journal of Cancer 59: 613–617

4. Spontaneous reporting

John C. C. Talbot

INTRODUCTION

A doctor describing his or her own clinical observations of a suspected adverse drug reaction (ADR) with a marketed drug is the basis of spontaneous or, as it is sometimes known, voluntary reporting. This reporting is dependent on the individual doctor's ability to recognize possible ADRs, link them to drug treatment and report their observations. Unlike reports received from clinical trials, spontaneous reports are unsolicited.

The publication of case reports of suspected ADRs in medical journals is an established way of alerting others to possible drug hazards. However, publication of case reports has many limitations because: only a small proportion can be published; many such reports are inadequately documented; publication depends on editorial idiosyncrasy, and there is considerable delay between a possible ADR occurring and the paper being published (see ch. 11).

Although published reports are important, the systematic schemes for collecting spontaneous reports which exist in drug regulatory authorities and pharmaceutical companies offer advantages. After the thalidomide tragedy most western countries established government-based schemes along the lines of the Committee on Safety of Medicines (CSM) yellow card system in Britain which started in 1964 (see chs. 8 and 9). More recently, most pharmaceutical companies have established databases of worldwide spontaneous reports with their products. These systems have a key advantage over publications because: these reports are accumulated over a period of time and from many sources; data are centralized; they can be standardized by the use of specially designed reporting forms, and dedicated professionals are available to assess and review them.

Case reports should include information about the patient

(demography and medical history), details of the suspect drug and other treatments (dose, route, duration and indication) and a description of the suspected ADR (symptoms and signs, timing, dechallenge and outcome). Additional information such as allergies, exclusion of alternative causes, drug blood levels, laboratory data and rechallenge are also helpful in the evaluation of individual spontaneous reports.

THE ROLE OF SPONTANEOUS REPORTING

Spontaneous reporting, unlike other surveillance techniques, is available immediately a new drug is marketed, continues indefinitely and covers the entire patient population receiving the drug. It is therefore the quickest way of identifying uncommon ADRs. Any doctor and, in some countries, other health care professionals and patients, can submit reports; this makes spontaneous reporting a potentially powerful tool. In practice, however it is unfortunate that many doctors choose never to report a suspected ADR. Spontaneous reporting can detect and characterize common reactions, perhaps confirming suspicions aroused during clinical trials with the drug, and identify rare reactions which pre-marketing studies with the drug cannot detect. Compared with large cohort or post-marketing surveillance studies it is also an inexpensive and highly cost effective method of surveillance. Spontaneous reporting is therefore the cornerstone of drug safety monitoring for marketed drugs.

Limitations of spontaneous reporting

One of the main disadvantages of any spontaneous reporting system is the gross under-reporting of possible ADRs. It has been estimated that between 1 and 10% only of cases are reported to the CSM, and it is likely that this range may be even greater, depending on the drug and the nature of the suspected reaction. Inman (1980) suggested that under-reporting was due to 'seven deadly sins': complacency, the mistaken belief that only safe drugs are allowed on the market; fear of litigation; guilt, because harm to the patient may have been caused by treatment; ambition to collect and publish a personal series of cases; ignorance of how to report; diffidence about reporting mere suspicions; and lethargy. The reasons for not reporting are undoubtedly complex.

Even when a decision to report is made doctors may delay completing forms perhaps because they lack time or because they are waiting for further information such as the outcome of the reaction or the exclusion of other possible causes. The quality of many case reports is also poor; in an attempt to improve this, companies and some regulatory authorities, e.g. the CSM, put considerable effort into designing suitable forms and following up important cases by letter, telephone and by using field workers. Some reports are unintentionally misleading in that another reason for the patient's symptoms or condition becomes apparent after the report was made. Again, careful investigation and longterm follow-up of cases should minimize this.

A major limitation of spontaneous reporting is the difficulty doctors have in recognizing previously unknown drug reactions. Some ADRs that are now well established were not immediately recognizable as such e.g. eye effects with β blockers or cough due to ACE inhibitors. Experience has shown that it often takes one or two astute doctors to make these initial observations before others submit similar reports. For example, it was not until the first cases of skin and eye reactions with the β blocker practolol were published that hundreds of reports were received by the CSM (Inman 1980) and ICI, leading to the worldwide withdrawal of the oral drug about a year after the initial publications.

Spontaneous reporting is a poor method of recognizing associations between drugs and events which commonly occur in the untreated population, identifying ADRs with a long latent period (particularly if the drug has been stopped) and events that are not usually thought of as being possible ADRs. It also lacks a control group, comparative information and denominator data which limit its role in confirming the existence of new ADRs.

What can and cannot be done with spontaneous reports

Occasionally, single or small numbers of spontaneous reports enable the recognition of a new ADR. This has usually been with typical acute recognized iatrogenic events, such as anaphylaxis occurring almost immediately after administration of the drug. Certain type A ADRs (ch. 1) can also be identified from spontaneous reports when reviewed in conjunction with an understanding of the pharmacology of the drug e.g. profound hypotension after starting a new antihypertensive drug. However, in most cases individual spontaneous reports only indicate suspicion of a new ADR, i.e. they generate a hypothesis, but do not usually confirm it.

In some instances, examination of a number of spontaneous reports by the regulatory authority or pharmaceutical company has led to the identification and characterization of an ADR, e.g. by showing a similar clinical presentation, time to onset or other feature. Examples of this process include pulmonary reactions with nitrofurantoin (Penn & Griffin 1982) and ketaconazole hepatotoxicity (Lake-Bakaar et al 1987). In others, particular risk factors have been identified, e.g. the susceptibility of children to sodium valproate fatal hepatotoxicity (Powell-Jackson et al 1984) and the higher frequency of metoclopramide-associated acute dystonic and dyskinetic reactions in adolescents, particularly females (Bateman et al 1985).

However, spontaneous reports do not usually prove a causal relationship between the drug and the ADR. This is particularly so where there is a background of the clinical condition in the patient population and where the ADR could mimic naturally occurring disease. In these situations hypotheses generated by spontaneous reports may be confirmed in two major ways (see ch. 3): firstly, by looking at populations of patients who did and did not receive the drug, i.e. experimental or observational cohort studies; and secondly, by examining whether patients with the event (and matched controls without the event) received the drug i.e. case-control studies. In other cases, hypotheses can be confirmed by special tests, e.g. skin testing, or by reference to the chemical structure or pharmacology of the drug. Table 4.1 gives examples of some ADRs identified by spontaneous reporting and subsequently confirmed by other means.

As indicated in chapter 1, spontaneous reports cannot give the incidence of an ADR. This is because neither the numerator (number of reports) nor the denominator (number of patients exposed) can be accurately known. ADRs are grossly underreported and there is no way of knowing what proportion of suspected reactions have been reported. Uncertainty also exists as to how many reports are actually drug-related and how many are due to another factor i.e. disease or other drugs. The denominator can be estimated from sales figures or numbers of prescriptions [Intercontinental Medical Statistics (IMS) or Prescribing Analysis and Costs (PACT) data], but since individual drugs are given in varying doses and for different durations in various indications, the estimates are usually very crude.

Table 4.1 Examples of ADRs identified by spontaneous reporting

Drug	Adverse drug reaction	Confirmed by
Stilboestrol	Vaginal adenocarcinoma in daughters	Case-control study
Practolol	Oculomucocutaneous syndrome	Skin testing and further reports
Oral contraceptives	Pulmonary embolism, myocardial infarction	MRC case-control studies
Halothane	Jaundice	Retrospective cohort study, large-scale randomized controlled trial
Chloramphenicol	Aplastic anaemia	Nationwide survey in USA
Phenylbutazone	Agranulocytosis, aplastic anaemia	Structural similarity to amidopyrine and other pyrazolones known to cause bone marrow toxicity

Adapted from Venning 1983

Incidence rates can be provided from clinical trials or other cohort studies but only apply to the population in that study. Case-control studies only provide a measure of relative risk, not absolute incidence figures. In reality the incidence of many ADRs varies enormously depending on the population receiving the drug. For instance, the incidence of a dose-dependent ADR in the elderly or in patients with renal impairment may be several times greater than the 'normal' adult population.

Comparing spontaneous reports with different drugs

It is attractive to think that the spontaneous reports received with one drug could be compared with those received with another, similar, drug. However, many biases affect the reporting of suspected ADRs, and one should be very cautious about drawing conclusions from such data. Despite possible biases some comparisons have shown important differences. Comparing reporting rates of ADRs with sales volumes, it was shown that the risk of Guillain-Barré syndrome and hepatotoxicity with zimeldine, and haemolytic anaemia and hepatotoxicity with nomifensine, were substantially greater than with other antidepressants and both drugs were withdrawn. Reporting rates of serious gastrointestinal suspected ADRs with non-steroidal anti-inflammatory drugs

(NSAIDs) in the UK showed essentially three categories (CSM 1986): (a) increased reporting, e.g. benoxaprofen, indoprofen, fenclofenac, feprazone and Osmosin which have all been withdrawn; (b) less reporting, e.g. ibuprofen which was made a pharmacy (P) medicine, available without a prescription but under a pharmacist's supervision; and (c) a group between these where the drugs remain as prescription only medicines (POM).

The comparison of reporting rates with drugs in the same therapeutic class falsely assumes that the same patient population receives the different drugs. For instance, any patient with asthma who must have a β blocker should be given a cardioselective drug such as atenolol rather than propranolol. Because of its greater use in this patient group more reports of bronchospasm associated with atenolol are received despite it being the safer drug in this respect. Furthermore, patients who have previously suffered ADRs with an older drug are likely to be given the new drug instead. Thus, patients who are most likely to experience ADRs tend to receive one drug rather than another.

Spontaneous reporting can provide reassurance about the safety of a drug. An absence of spontaneous reports alone does not prove safety but an absence of serious reports with a widely used drug is very reassuring. The change in status of some medicines from POM to P e.g. ibuprofen, loperamide and more recently mebendazole, was made partly on the evidence gained from spontaneous reporting.

FACTORS INFLUENCING SPONTANEOUS REPORTING

As already stated, there is considerable under-reporting of many ADRs and reporting is influenced by several factors. The number of reports is clearly linked to the sales or use of the drug. Large numbers of reports have been received with some relatively safe drugs because of their widespread use e.g. H2 antagonists, cimetidine and ranitidine.

Reporting rates are also a function of how long the drug has been on the market, with the highest reporting occurring in the first few years. This leads to the detection of new ADRs, which is good, but doctors then no longer submit reports as they are seen as recognized effects. This can be short-sighted as the extent of the problem may have initially been under-estimated and further reports may enable the reaction to be better characterized. Reporting is also influenced by the side-effect profile of other similar drugs. The fact that a particular ADR is recognized with an earlier drug of the same type encourages doctors to report instances with the new drug which can bias its ADR profile. ADR reporting can also increase sharply when attention is drawn to specific problems with the drug, similar drugs or drug safety issues in general. This was seen with practolol and other β blockers in the mid-1970s and benoxaprofen and other NSAIDs in the early 1980s. Reporting may also be affected by the interplay between the seriousness of the suspected ADR and the seriousness of the condition being treated.

SOURCE OF SPONTANEOUS REPORTS

Spontaneous reports received by regulatory authorities and pharmaceutical companies come from many sources including doctors, pharmacists, nurses, published literature, coroners, lawyers and patients directly.

In the UK the CSM only accepts reports from doctors although there are a number of schemes in which hospital pharmacists encourage reporting (Veitch & Talbot 1985). Around 70% of reports received by the CSM are from general practitioners who clearly play a vital role in this form of monitoring. About 15% of Yellow Cards are from hospital doctors; although a much smaller proportion, these are often the most serious suspected reactions such as haematological or hepatic reactions, perhaps causing death, admission to hospital or the need for specialist management. In reality a relatively small group of doctors report more frequently and probably over half have never sent a report. This is most unsatisfactory and the system would be much improved if more doctors actively participated. The remaining 15% of reports to the CSM come from pharmaceutical companies.

In some other countries pharmacists can also report suspected ADRs to the local regulatory authority e.g. Ireland and Australia, and in the USA the Food and Drug Administration (FDA) accepts reports from any source. About 90% of reports to the FDA come from the pharmaceutical industry in contrast to the reporting pattern in Britain.

Pharmaceutical companies receive most spontaneous reports from doctors, hospital pharmacists and via their company representatives. Reporters often enquire whether the suspected reaction has been seen before, indicating that companies are regarded as an important information source on ADRs.

OBLIGATIONS OF PHARMACEUTICAL COMPANIES

Companies are concerned about the safety of the medicines they market and monitor spontaneous reports from many sources as an alert to new problems and to characterize recognized ADRs. In addition, companies have to report certain ADRs to the regulatory authorities in countries where the drug is sold (see ch. 9).

Company databases

Most major pharmaceutical companies now use computerized databases to handle their spontaneous reports. If the UK company is a subsidiary of a foreign-based international company (usually US, Swiss or German) the UK database may be relatively small, even on one personal computer. However, major British companies such as Glaxo, ICI and Wellcome all have large computerized international databases of spontaneous reports. Subsidiary companies send details of local spontaneous reports to company headquarters where they are added to a central database. This may be done by directly entering the data into the central database via a foreign subsidiary, or by updating from a disc or manually. The current Glaxo central database has direct entry from both the UK and Glaxo Inc. in the USA, with reports from other countries being sent to and entered in the UK (Talbot 1989). In future, further remote data entry facilities are planned.

The number of spontaneous reports received by the major pharmaceutical companies worldwide is considerable. Computer systems are needed simply to handle and track these numbers of case reports. However, the main function of such systems is the identification of hypotheses and characterization of new ADRs. These databases can be used to answer specific questions from doctors and pharmacists which, in some cases, may influence patient management. In this way companies provide a useful information source, but the provision of this requires reports to be sent in the first place. Companies certainly have more resources to provide such information than the regulatory authority staff.

The sophisticated computer systems in existence can generate the reporting forms for the regulatory authorities (see ch. 9); they can also present data in tabular or graphic form to facilitate identification of risk factors for the ADR such as age, sex, other drugs, underlying disease etc. (see ch. 7).

The main advantage of company databases is that they are international, hence the database may be larger than that of the regulatory authority and include data from more reporters. In some instances drugs may be marketed in other countries before the UK and reports from these countries are a useful information source. Another advantage of some company databases is that they are more sophisticated and powerful than some regulatory authority databases and can be searched more quickly and produce better outputs and analyses.

CONCLUSION

Spontaneous reporting is the cornerstone of drug safety monitoring after a drug is marketed. It can identify certain new reactions and generate hypotheses that may be confirmed by other methods. It can help characterize certain ADRs and identify patients at risk. Spontaneous reporting does, however, have limitations, in particular the difficulty in recognizing some reactions and the underreporting of cases.

Pharmaceutical companies welcome spontaneous reports with their products. They are obliged to forward details of certain cases to the CSM and some overseas regulatory authorities. Companies use their worldwide databases to provide an information service to doctors and pharmacists, to generate new hypotheses and to characterize ADRs.

REFERENCES

Bateman D N, Rawlins M D, Simpson J M 1985 Extrapyramidal reactions with metoclopramide. British Medical Journal 291: 930–932
CSM 1986 CSM Update: Non-steroidal anti-inflammatory drugs and serious gastrointestinal adverse reactions 2. British Medical Journal 292: 1190–1191
Inman W H W 1980 Monitoring for drug safety. MTP Press, Lancaster, pp36–37.
Lake-Bakaar G, Scheuer P J, Sherlock S 1987 Hepatic reactions associated with ketoconazole in the United Kingdom. British Medical Journal 294: 419–422
Penn R G, Griffin J P 1982 Adverse reactions to nitrofurantoin in the United Kingdom, Sweden and Holland. British Medical Journal 284: 1440–1442
Powell-Jackson P R, Tredger J M, Williams R 1984 Hepatotoxicity to sodium valproate: a review. Gut 25: 673–681
Talbot J C C 1989 Database management and reporting systems – foreign-based companies: The Glaxo approach. Drug Information Journal 23: 189–196.
Veitch G B A, Talbot J C C 1985 The pharmacist and adverse drug reaction reporting. Pharmaceutical Journal 234: 107–109.
Venning G R 1983 Identification of adverse reactions to new drugs. II – How were 18 important adverse reactions discovered and with what delays? British Medical Journal 286: 289–292, 365–368

5. Has the patient suffered an ADR? – assessment of drug causality

M. D. B. Stephens

INTRODUCTION

Many ordinary people not taking any medication or suffering from any illness will, if asked, admit to symptoms – had they been taking a medicine, they might have blamed it as the cause of their symptoms. A survey of students and university staff found that 80% of them fell into this category (Reidenberg & Lowenthal 1968).

Some very sensitive patients appear to feel normal physiological processes to the extent that they mistake them for signs of disease. When these are added to the burden of symptoms caused by acute or chronic disease it sometimes becomes difficult to separate the 'wheat' from the 'chaff'.

When a patient thinks that a medicine 'doesn't agree with them', 'is not suiting them' or 'is upsetting them' then the doctor may reply 'I'm sorry to hear that. How is it affecting you?' The doctor may recognize the symptoms as a possible side-effect of the drug or if not he or she will probably turn to the Monthly Index of Medical Specialities (MIMS) for help. If there is no support there for a drug-induced effect the doctor will rarely contradict the patient. If needs be, a different medicine will be prescribed, without knowing whether or not the drug had definitely caused the event. Probably only if the patient presents as a continuing problem or is seriously disturbed by the event will the doctor take the matter further, either by prescribing a medicine for the potential adverse reaction (after having stopped the previous medicine) or by undertaking further investigations.

Life is too short to decide whether or not every symptom is definitely caused by a medicine; but doctors may, when next they see the manufacturer's representative, mention it in passing. I hope that the representative will then take down the details of the event on the company's adverse event (AE) form and send it back to the company drug surveillance department for assessment. How can the prescribing doctor or the company staff assess whether or not there has been an adverse drug reaction (ADR)? What are the mechanisms of drug-induced reactions?

MECHANISM OF ADRs

An ADR may occur because it is a feature of the drug's pharmacology, i.e. type A, and will increase in severity as the dose is increased; again, since it is linked with the pharmacological action it will tend to occur in a large proportion of the population, e.g. dry mouth with tricyclic antidepressants, headaches with vasodilators. Luckily, many of these reactions regress as the body adapts to them. Most doctors are aware, from their own experience as well as from basic pharmacological knowledge, of the type A ADRs associated with their own favourite drugs. These type A ADRs are then the drugs' 'fault', whilst the type B ADRs are the patients' 'fault' because some peculiarity of the patient has made them become hypersensitive to the drug.

The type B ADR will not be predictable since it is not related to the known pharmacology of the drug. These type B reactions may mimic almost any sort of natural disease, from urticaria to Guillain-Barré syndrome. Those natural diseases with allergic or immunological abnormalities are perhaps more frequently mimicked by drugs than others, but this is very unpredictable and if the onset of symptoms occurs some time after starting a drug then the association may be missed by the prescribing doctor.

DETECTION OF ADRs

The pre-marketing clinical trials should have discovered the most common type A ADR in the restricted population recruited in these studies; however, many subgroups will have been excluded from the trial protocols, e.g. children and the very elderly. In the post-marketing period further clinical trials will be undertaken to delineate the use of the drug.

After marketing, the use of the drug will not be monitored so strictly, and spotting the more rare ADR will be dependent on the alertness of the practising physician. Individual clinicians have always been the most productive source of new hypotheses concerning ADRs. This is especially true if, by being very specialized, a lot of very similar patients pass through their hands, or one or two drugs are prescribed frequently in their practice.

Since ADRs act through the same physiological and pathological pathways as normal disease they are difficult, and sometimes impossible, to distinguish. The numbers of ADRs which have no equivalent natural disease must be very few, e.g. the practolol-induced syndrome, whereas there are many which are, in themselves, indistinguishable from the natural disease, e.g. pulmonary embolism with the oral contraceptive. The differential diagnosis of most diseases includes the consideration of drugs as a possible factor.

Differential diagnosis

Any differences between the natural disease and the drug-induced disease can be used in differential diagnosis but the main factors are:

1. The time interval between taking the drug and the first appearance of the signs and/or symptoms of the AE.
2. The time interval between stopping the drug and the disappearance of the AE or, in some cases, the continuation of the AE despite stopping the drug. This is generally known as the response to dechallenge.
3. If the drug is given on a subsequent occasion it is referred to as a rechallenge and the AE may or may not recur.
4. The known record of the drug.
5. Alternative causes of the AE.
6. Any specific laboratory tests.

Let us consider each of these factors in some detail.

The time to onset

The time to onset of a type A reaction will depend on the pharmacokinetics of the drug and the tissue threshold necessary for the reaction. For an oral drug this will probably be between half an hour and the time to reach steady state (five times the half life of the drug). For intravenous drugs the onset may be instantaneous.

Type B reactions require a minimum of 5 days on treatment before the cells become hypersensitive to the drug but there is no maximum time for these reactions to have occurred (although most will have occurred by 12 weeks). However, some may be delayed as long as a year, e.g. tardive dyskinesia with neuroleptics. This longer time to onset means that sometimes the reaction appears after the drug has been stopped, e.g. agranulocytosis.

The response to dechallenge

Again, type A reactions disappear according to pharmacokinetic principles – usually the tissue level falls quickly below the threshold level, but it depends on whether tissue damage has occurred. Tissue damage may be permanent and therefore the reaction may be irreversible. If the doctor recognizes the event as a type A ADR he or she may reduce the dosage until the ADR disappears and then check whether it is efficacious enough for that patient.

Type B reactions usually respond more slowly, and again the proviso of tissue damage applies.

Frequently, the situation is confounded by a further drug either being substituted for the offending drug or being used as therapy for the AE.

Rechallenge

A rechallenge may be accidental or deliberate. In the former, previous use may not have caused a reaction or, if it did so, the event may not have been recognized as the result of treatment. The most common form of rechallenge is when the AE occurs soon after taking the drug and has worn off before the next dose is due, so that the patient complains of the event occurring every time the drug is taken. Sometimes the previous reaction has been forgotten by the patient or has not been recorded by the doctor. A deliberate rechallenge is sometimes undertaken when the use of that particular drug is thought to be essential for the patient. Most commonly, if the reaction has been type A, the rechallenge starts with a small dose and is then gradually increased until the first sign of the reaction appears. This approach may enable the patient to benefit from the drug without any adverse effect. If the reaction has no objective signs the doctor may wish to rechallenge the patient by using a placebo and active drug in a blinded fashion.

On the whole, type B reactions are not rechallenged because any subsequent reaction may be very much more serious than the original reaction and might have a fatal outcome.

The decision to rechallenge depends on several factors, the most important of which is the avoidance of any permanent harm to the patient. If a type A ADR is thought to have occurred and it was completely reversible in a very short time without inconveniencing the patient too much, a doctor may consider rechallenging the patient (Stephens 1983). This decision will depend largely on the risks associated with any alternative treatments and how great is the suspicion that the drug caused the original event.

Is it a known reaction to the drug?

The main known ADRs to a drug should be listed in the data sheet and in the ABPI compendium. All the known ADRs are published in the latest edition of Meyler's *Side-effects of Drugs* and the *Side-effects of Drugs Annual*. But there is frequently a long delay between the diagnosis of a new ADR and its first publication, the mean delay being over a year (Haramburu et al 1985), so the delay is even longer for these secondary publications. For more up-to-date information one can turn to the journal *Reactions Weekly*, but this is obviously not available to most doctors. First of all help should be sought from a pharmacist, either a retail pharmacist or a hospital pharmacist; the latter will have access to either books or ADR databases, and if more up-to-date advice is required the drug company will frequently be contacted.

Alternative causes of the event

Many minor AEs similar to minor drug-associated events also occur frequently in normal life without any obvious cause, but more serious ADRs may mimic any natural disease. One must also consider other drug and non-drug treatments. The chances of developing an ADR vary directly with the number of drugs taken including, of course, over-the-counter drugs and herbal medicines and this accounts for the increase in ADRs in the elderly. The possibility of interaction must always be kept in mind.

Any specific laboratory tests

Laboratory tests may include blood drug levels, antibody tests and lymphocyte toxicity assays – in fact any test that can help differentiate drug cause and natural disease.

All six factors influencing differential diagnosis are then considered with the other known facts of the case in order to reach a diagnosis. This mental process has been called 'global intro-spection'.

METHODS OF CAUSALITY ASSESSMENT

Several groups of clinical pharmacologists have examined 'global introspection' as a method for diagnosis. By having a set of different cases diagnosed by several different experts they have found that the level of disagreement is very high. Various methods have been put forward to obtain better agreement. These formal methods have included defined criteria, algorithms and visual analogue scales.

Defined criteria are used by the Swedish and Australian regulatory authorities. The Australian definition of 'certain' is, for example, 'confirmed by rechallenge and/or confirmed by laboratory data and/or plausible, reaction immediately (within 5 minutes) following administration'. Most drug companies use an algorithm or 'global introspection'. An algorithm can be defined in this context as a formalized procedure to process in a step-wise fashion the information about a single AE in order to identify an ADR as such and to assess the possibility of a true drug–AE relationship. In all, 23 methods have been published by three groups of physicians (Stephens 1987):

1. Clinicians (10)
2. Regulatory authorities (6)
3. Pharmaceutical industry physicians (7).

The clinician often does not need to make a positive diagnosis of an ADR since if they or the patient feel that the drug is causing problems they can usually simply stop the drug and, if necessary, substitute an alternative treatment. It has been the clinical pharmacologists who have taken most interest in producing more formal methods of diagnosis.

The regulatory authorities have special requirements; since they are inundated with reports, any method must be quick to apply and simple. The method would have to be suitable for use with minimal data and have an explanatory capacity. Overall it would need to be sensitive rather than specific. The regulatory authorities have responded in different ways to this challenge; the American and UK authorities have given up using their methods and now do not use a particular method of diagnosis, whilst the French specify their own method for use both by themselves and the pharmaceutical industry.

The pharmaceutical industry has the most stringent demands on any method of diagnosis:

1. It must be sensitive and specific. If it is not sensitive it will be accused of bias by its critics, but at the same time it is important that 'wolf' is not cried unnecessarily.
2. It must be able to use every bit of information available. The industry usually has both the time and the staff to acquire further information and occasionally hospital records are made available.
3. It must balance the possibilities of drug cause and non-drug cause for each factor. The majority of the algorithms do not do this but use alternative causes as an additional factor as described above. There are two exceptions: one method uses the equivalent of an analogue scale for each factor with drug cause and non-drug cause at opposite ends (see Fig.5.1) but fails to meet other criteria; the second method [Bayesian Adverse Reaction Diagnostic Instrument (BARDI)] will be described later in this chapter.
4. Important information should be able to over-rule neutral information. Again, many algorithms fail in this respect.
5. It must have an explanatory capacity. A physician assessing drug-associated AEs within the industry will need considerable integrity if he or she is to resist the pressure from colleagues to find 'their' drug innocent. It is therefore imperative that the method used entails a written explanation of the causality assessment.
6. It must be rapid for cases with minimal data. The majority of cases reaching industry will not have complete records of drugs used, laboratory tests, etc. A large company is likely to receive as many AE reports as the regulatory authorities do in many small countries.

There is no one method of diagnosis that can meet all these criteria; the nearest is the BARDI method which meets all but the last criterion. Bayes' theorem requires that one balances the odds between the drug causing the event and there being an alternative cause for that type of AE before the event in question occurred; this is called the 'prior odds'. The 'prior odds' is then multiplied by the 'likelihood ratio', which is a balancing of the factors for the present event between the drug causing it and there being an

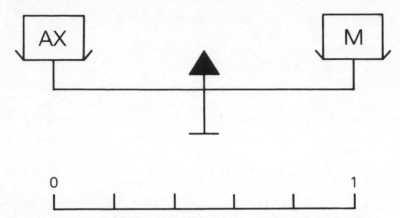

Fig. 5.1   Analogue scale for drug cause and non-drug cause. AX, Alternative explanation; M, Medication (After Lagier et al 1983)

alternative cause, e.g. disease. This may be a lengthy process requiring literature searches for previous surveys and studies. So at present the industry needs to use 'global introspection' or an algorithm for the non-controversial cases, and BARDI for those AEs which are controversial and/or are of vital importance.

In order to have the best chance of deciding whether or not a drug caused an AE it is important to collect any evidence that has a bearing on the case. The company AE form is designed to collect the essential data and then, depending on its nature, the company may request further information from the reporting doctor (see ch. 8). The company form should also ask the doctor's opinion as to whether the drug caused the event since he or she will know the patient and the disease, whilst the company physician will know the drug and probably have had more experience in assessment of these cases.

The opinion requested should not be a yes or no answer but should give sufficient alternatives such that the reporting doctor is not forced one way or the other. Since it is hardly ever possible to say whether an event is or is not definitely caused by the drug, these absolute terms should be avoided. The reporting doctor is under no obligation either to fill in the company's form or to give the company any information, so the pharmaceutical industry is very beholden to the prescriber. Any information given by the doctors is, of course, not identified with a name or NHS number and should be strictly anonymous.

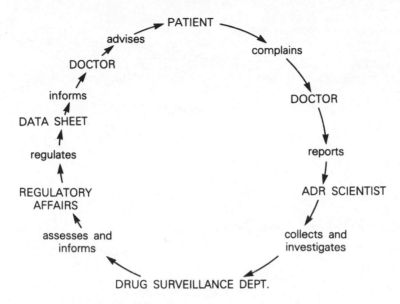

Fig. 5.2 Information chain for adverse drug reactions (ADRs)

Using the information provided by the prescriber about the patient, the underlying disease and the AE, and adding this to the knowledge of the drug from the company, the company physician can make a diagnosis which is then added to the database. If the originating physician has asked any questions about whether there have been any other similar reports or whether the company thought that the event could have been caused by the drug, then a reply will be sent back thanking them and answering these questions. Periodic surveys of the database will often lead to the decision that an AE is caused by the drug and a recommendation made that it should be included in the data sheet for the benefit of the prescriber and the patient (ch. 7). The ultimate benefit to the patient depends on all concerned taking their responsibilities seriously. The chain is only as strong as its weakest link (Fig. 5.2). Please don't let that weak link be you.

REFERENCES

Haramburu F, Begaud B, Pere J C, Marcel S, Albin H 1985 Role of medical journals in ADR alerts. Lancet 2 September 2: 550–551
Lagier G, Vincens M, Castol A 1983 Imputabilité en pharmacovigilance principe de la méthode appreciative pondéré (MAP) et principals erreurs a éviter. Therapie 38: 308–318

Reidenberg M M, Lowenthal D T 1968 Adverse nondrug reactions. New England
  Journal of Medicine 279: 678–679
Stephens M D B 1983 Deliberate drug rechallenge. Human Toxicology 2: 573–
  577
Stephens M D B 1987 The diagnosis of adverse medical events associated with
  drug treatment. Adverse Drug Reaction Acute Poisoning Review 1: 1–35

6. The interface between the medical profession and the pharmaceutical industry

Elliot G. Brown

As has been discussed in chapter 4, the doctor who prescribes a drug and observes its effects in the patient is in a unique position to raise the suspicion of a previously unrecognized adverse reaction. There may also be a need on the part of the doctor to obtain information about safety aspects of a particular drug in greater detail than can be found simply by looking in a standard text or by reading a data sheet. The pharmaceutical manufacturer, on the other hand, needs to know about possible new hazards with its products and may have available the detailed information on safety which the doctor seeks. There are, however, barriers to the free exchange of information between the doctor and the pharmaceutical company; some of these are real and some are matters of perception. This chapter intends to explore some of the issues; much of the material covered is dependent on individual viewpoint, but it is hoped that an even-handed approach has been adopted.

The first question to be considered relates to the reasons why pharmaceutical companies wish to know about the doctor's suspicions about an adverse reaction and what advantages there are for the doctor in liaising with the company. Consideration is then given to some of the difficulties that exist which may prevent this intercourse, ethical problems, medicolegal issues, and some perceptual barriers.

The subject of the next part of the chapter is whether the pharmaceutical industry can offer any safeguards and reassurances that it will handle reports of adverse reactions appropriately. What constitute reasonable expectations regarding the way the company deals with the report, and indeed what the company can reasonably expect of the reporting doctor, is then addressed.

As was stated earlier, much of the following discussion depends on individual point of view but certain topics are particularly open to debate in relation to the reporting of adverse reactions in general;

the final part of this chapter will look at some of these areas of controversy.

REASONS FOR REPORTING SUSPECTED ADVERSE REACTIONS TO MANUFACTURERS

The pharmaceutical company needs to know about the safety of its products to ensure that precautions in use and warnings about potential hazards of its drugs can be adequately communicated to prescribing doctors. The company also has to keep the regulatory authorities informed of new or serious adverse reactions (ADRs), so that the medical profession and the public can be assured that the benefit–risk analysis is constantly being reviewed by disinterested parties. Whilst information about ADRs reported directly by doctors to regulatory authorities, such as the Committee on Safety of Medicines (CSM), is passed on to the manufacturer, such information may be delayed and incomplete. Direct reporting to the company by the doctor allows relevant details about the case to be established.

There are advantages to the doctor in reporting to the pharmaceutical company. The company holds published and unpublished information about its drugs. It can advise on whether a reaction has been seen previously with its product, on previous experience of management of a problem, and on its outcome. The company may help the doctor with literature searches, and may assist with the writing and publication of case reports. It may also help by providing specially formulated drugs for double-blind rechallenge, or by providing access to specialized laboratory services for assay of blood levels of drug or other special tests.

Despite the advantages to the doctor which might result from contacting the pharmaceutical company, and the benefits which accrue to the company, there are several reasons why doctors who suspect an adverse reaction choose not to contact the company, electing either to report directly to a regulatory body or not to report at all.

BARRIERS TO REPORTING ADVERSE REACTIONS DIRECTLY TO MANUFACTURERS

Ethical dilemmas

Doctors who suspect an adverse reaction to a particular drug may feel that the patient's trust is being betrayed, and particularly that confidentiality is compromised, if the reaction is reported to a third party. There are additional implications because the manufacturer has a commercial interest in the effects of the drug. The doctor may also have reservations about the way the company will handle the information provided. There may be concern that non-professional or unqualified persons might make improper use of this: that the information could appear on databases which could be accessed externally. The doctor may have doubts about the behaviour of a particular company in other areas, for example in the marketing of its products or in dealing with claims for damages by patients.

Medicolegal issues

In the UK, there is no legal or other requirement for doctors to report adverse reactions; in some countries, e.g. France, reporting to the regulatory authority is mandatory. The doctor may be anxious that the information which is to be reported could be used in a court of law to his or her disadvantage, for example as an admission of liability in a civil case alleging negligence. Conversely, there may be concern that by reporting the ADR to the company, the doctor might in some way compromise the patient's case if damages were to be claimed against the manufacturer.

Other barriers to reporting

The doctor may decide that it is unnecessary to duplicate a report of the adverse reaction by reporting to both the CSM and the pharmaceutical company. To some extent, the doctor may feel exposed to criticism from the company for the way that the clinical problem has been handled. The doctor may fear that the company will bother him or her with repeated requests for detailed information, or that the company may unreasonably deny the possibility of its products causing harm. If the doctor is considering publication of a case report, he or she may worry that the company might apply coercion to try to prevent this from happening.

Chapter 4 mentions some of the reasons why doctors may not report adverse reactions to the CSM, some of these reasons may apply to reporting to companies also.

However, are these justifiable doubts and fears on the part of the medical profession? Are there other dimensions to the ethical question, and what safeguards exist if doctors report directly to the company?

SAFEGUARDS AND REASSURANCES

It is certainly the case that companies are interested to receive reports of adverse reactions, even if reports have been made to the regulatory authority. As regards the ethical dilemma, the basis of the trust which a patient places in the doctor is the belief that the doctor will always do what is best for that individual. However, it is recognized that the greater public good may have to be taken into account on occasion, economic constraints may be applied, or actions may have to be prioritized on the basis of greater need by other patients and limited resources. Implicit in the doctor–patient relationship is the need for confidentiality but, again, this is sometimes waived in the public interest or in a court of law.

A factor to be taken into account in reporting suspected adverse reactions to the manufacturer is that future patients may benefit if the information helps the company to quantify the hazards associated with use of the drug. Of more direct benefit to the patient concerned, the company may be able to advise about other similar reports and thereby make diagnosis and management more straightforward. Moreover, the identity of the individual patient need not be disclosed to the company, although some form of identification is necessary to avoid duplication of reporting unless it is made clear that the CSM has also been informed.

Improper behaviour on the part of the pharmaceutical industry in this context could occur, but two factors which prevent this are the functional division of pharmaceutical companies into separate marketing and medical departments, and the recognition of the serious damage done to a company when its ethical reputation is tarnished. Adverse publicity about unethical behaviour by a company is extremely damaging and can affect its product marketing, the willingness of doctors to perform clinical trials with its drugs and of patients to participate in them, and the ability of the company to recruit and retain high-calibre staff.

Reports of ADRs are handled by the company's medical department; a registered medical practitioner is directly involved in the process, or has responsibility for delegating this function to others under his or her supervision.

The company doctor is subject to the same code of ethics and is accountable to his or her professional peers in the same way as any other doctor; it is the company doctor's responsibility to ensure that no information about the reporting doctor or the patient is made available inappropriately, and that no direct approaches would be made to the patient.

Security of documents and computers is enforced and strict confidentiality is maintained within the company, subject to fulfilling legal requirements for reporting to regulatory authorities. There is no requirement for any patient to be directly identifiable in documentation or computer file by name or address.

With regard to medicolegal implications of reporting adverse reactions, provided the doctor does not directly attribute blame to him or herself in the report, there should be no risk directly resulting from reporting the reaction in the event of litigation by the patient. There have, however, been occasional reports of a doctor fraudulently reporting an AE as part of bogus participation in a clinical trial for which he is receiving payment. Charges of fraud and professional misconduct may ensue.

If a doctor has prescribed a medicine in good faith, in accordance with the data sheet and with appropriate care, successful litigation is unlikely in response to adverse reactions. However, the doctor must accept full responsibility for taking all due care with his prescription, and must consider whether the patient should be warned of any hazard. According to the doctrine sometimes called 'strict liability', recent UK law makes the manufacturer liable if the medicine is defective, i.e. causes an adverse reaction which was not identified and notified to the prescriber before the time of prescribing. The company could have a defence if there was no way in which it could have anticipated this in advance. There is no requirement to show that the company is negligent, only that injury has resulted from the defect. In any case, whether or not the doctor reported the occurrence of a suspected adverse reaction to the company would have no impact on the legal considerations regarding product liability or negligence. The doctor may be legally liable if he has prescribed the drug without taking appropriate care, and damage resulted, but there is no liability devolving on the prescriber simply because an adverse reaction occurred, if he has not been negligent.

Increasingly, the patient is being brought into the prescribing decision. Led by European Community legislation, pharmaceutical companies are giving product information directly to patients in package leaflets. The prescriber may prescribe without warning the patient about side-effects, but it is foreseeable that one day a prescriber could be held to be negligent for failing to give such a warning before prescribing.

It is the case, however, that the report of a doctor to the pharmaceutical company is 'discoverable' in law, and may be required by a court to be made available to the parties in an action.

If the doctor feels that he can overcome the various 'obstacles' to direct reporting to the company, what should he expect in his dealings with the company? In turn, what can the company expect of the doctor?

EXPECTATIONS

Reporting doctors have a right to expect the following from the pharmaceutical company:

1. Observations should be received with interest and courtesy
2. Confidentiality of the individual patient should be maintained
3. The response should be non-judgmental
4. Information should be professionally evaluated and appropriate action taken
5. Information from the company to the doctor in response should be non-promotional, even-handed and accurately reflect current knowledge
6. Requests for further details, whether by telephone, letter or at a follow-up visit should be relevant and the doctor's time must be respected.

In turn, the company may have the following expectations:

1. The doctor will act responsibly in reporting, reports being legible and comprehensible and as complete as possible
2. If the doctor is making a serious allegation about the drug's safety, sufficient evidence will be provided to allow the evaluation of the problem
3. The doctor will extend courtesy to professional staff from the company who are seeking appropriate information.

As was pointed out in the introduction to this chapter, opinions differ on many of these issues, but some areas stimulate particular debate. It is pertinent to consider these in the light of what has already been said.

CONTROVERSIES

In the whole area of the relationship between doctors, patients and the pharmaceutical industry, there is much that is contentious. An adversarial position is often adopted, with consumer groups, the medical and allied professions, government and the media all drawn into (sometimes acrimonious) debate. The controversies raised in this chapter are less often aired, but are still important and interesting. Hopefully, they are open to a more considered approach than sometimes applies.

Direct reporting by non-medically qualified persons

Anybody is free to report their suspicions about an adverse reaction directly to a pharmaceutical company or to the regulatory authority. In some countries, such as the USA, reports by patients, nurses, pharmacists and others are given similar consideration to those made by a doctor. In these countries, pharmaceutical companies are required to forward such non-medically confirmed reports to the regulatory authority, according to the same criteria as for reports by doctors. In other countries, including the UK and many European countries, it is only the medically confirmed suspected adverse reaction which is forwarded to the regulatory authority by the company, although other reports will be recorded and may be included in tabulations and analyses.

The arguments in favour of direct reporting by patients include the possibility that, in this way, multiple reports of previously unrecognized hazards could come to light at a relatively early time after marketing a new drug. However, this sensitivity is clearly at the expense of specificity, and the majority of such patient reports are for minor problems, often unrelated to the medicine. A higher degree of specificity in reporting applies to reports from health care professionals other than doctors. However, it is sometimes the case that, when these reports are followed up with the patient's doctor, the doctor is satisfied that the drug is not implicated; there are other factors, of which the reporter was unaware (e.g. concomitant medication or intercurrent illness) which provide a more feasible explanation for the observed event. Nevertheless, the potential of such reports as an alerting system has to be recognized. A possible area for concern in the reporting of AEs by individuals other than the patient's own doctor, is the risk of undermining the doctor-patient relationship. Clearly, considerable sensitivity and tact need to be exercised by the recipients of these reports in ensuring that conflict between doctor and patient or other health professional is not engendered.

Payment for adverse reaction reporting

The reporting of a suspected adverse reaction to a pharmaceutical company requires little effort and time on the part of the doctor; in the first instance a phone call, a brief note or copy of a hospital letter, or a photocopy of the report made to the regulatory authority (like the CSM 'Yellow Card'), may suffice. However, considerable time may be required in acceding to a company's subsequent request for detailed information. The Royal College of Physicians takes the view that reporting adverse reactions is part of normal professional activity, and does not warrant additional payment. Doctors are often prepared to spend the requisite time to provide follow-up information if they feel that the case is interesting, that the company is behaving responsibly, and that the welfare of patients as a whole is being served. However, it is not known to what extent under-reporting of adverse reactions results from unwillingness to perform additional work for no apparent recompense. There is a clear requirement that pharmaceutical companies should provide report forms which are straightforward to complete, and that they should be considerate in requesting additional detailed information, limiting this to essentials and to important cases.

The actions taken by pharmaceutical companies in response to reports of adverse reactions

The criticism is sometimes levelled at the pharmaceutical industry that it does not respond appropriately to reports of adverse reactions by suitable inclusion of statements in data sheets, especially in the contraindications, warnings, precautions and side-effects sections. It has been argued that companies are over-protective towards their products and are reluctant to add new warnings about possible hazards, or do not describe them adequately or in terms which are useful to the practising doctor. If doctors believed this to be the case, it would be a serious barrier to reporting suspicions of adverse reactions to a company's products.

There are several reasons why the company may not respond to reports of adverse reactions by including a statement in the data sheet. Commercial considerations should not come in to play here, but it sometimes happens that the manufacturer of a competitor product with the same actual adverse reaction profile does not make mention of a particular ADR, and therefore there may be some disadvantage in making reference to the reaction. In this context, if the reaction is an important one, it is likely that the regulatory authority will require inclusion of a suitable statement in all relevant data sheets. In some cases, there is a fine balance which has to be achieved in informing the prescribing doctor appropriately about ADRs, whilst not stopping him from using the drug in favour of a less safe preparation whose ADRs are less fully described, or a less effective preparation for the treatment of a potentially fatal condition. Some of the problems which companies face in this area of assessing reports of adverse reactions and communicating risk to doctors are discussed in chapter 7.

CONCLUSION

We have discussed the various aspects of the interface between the doctor who suspects an ADR and the pharmaceutical company which manufactured the drug. Whilst barriers do exist, there are advantages to both the doctor and the manufacturer if reporting is carried out and handled properly. The final consideration, however, must be the wellbeing of patients who are receiving the drug, whether it is the individual patient experiencing a suspected adverse reaction, or future patients who may benefit from knowledge adduced from the experience of others.

7. An overview of the role of industry

Win Castle

It is clear from previous chapters that the responsibility for the safety of medicines must be shared. However, industry plays a central role; employees, particularly pharmacists and doctors, exercise this responsibility on behalf of the company. The responsibility for drug safety is an interesting and important challenge and the purpose of this chapter is to outline the general approach taken. It has been said that 'Inside every large problem there is a small problem trying to get out'. The fact that it is not an easy problem makes the work absorbing.

WHY DOES INDUSTRY MONITOR THE SAFETY OF ITS DRUGS?

- It is not to avoid paying compensation, although every statement about the safety of its medicines that industry makes has obvious implications.
- It is not to prevent a 'trial by media' where journalists pursue a possible lead (which is their job) to make a 'story'. If a potential safety issue is first leaked through the media it can cause tremendous problems for patients as well as their pharmacists and the medical profession. This is particularly true if the facts are not completely accurate. Patients taking the medicine may become alarmed and may not have immediate access to their general practitioners who can advise them.
- It is not only because the regulators require industry to monitor the safety of its medicines.
- Responsible industry monitors the safety of its drugs primarily to help doctors prescribe them safely to their patients, and it has an advantage over national regulatory authorities in that it receives worldwide information much more quickly than a local regulatory agency.

In summary, industry monitors the safety of its medicines so that it can quickly identify any new medical risks for the patients. Then, in collaboration with the regulatory authorities, industry should provide the best medical advice to health care professionals worldwide. If the health of patients is compromised rather than improved because of medical treatment all the different parties suffer. Nobody gains if the media takes it upon itself to pre-empt the rest of us in alerting the patients and their doctors to a supposed safety problem. Remember Murphy's law – if anything can go wrong it will.

SOURCES OF DATA FOR THE INDUSTRY

Industry receives reports on its drugs from five main sources:

1. Its tightly controlled clinical trials
2. Large uncontrolled observational surveys (see ch. 3)
3. Separate interesting cases reported from the 'market-place', where patients are prescribed the medicines outside the rigorous constraints of clinical trials
4. Some case reports originally presented in the published literature
5. Some reports passed on to industry from the regulatory authorities.

No information is completely ignored; for example, letters from consumers which are not medically substantiated are taken into account, although it is important to follow these up to get as much clinical detail as possible.

All the available information is stored in the databases of the industry because all sources must be reviewed to monitor effectively the safety of the medicines. Unfortunately, all these data cannot be added together mathematically because the different sources of information inherently give different slants to the problem, and the amount of information and its reliability can vary markedly. This is the addendum to Murphy's law: 'In precise mathematical terms $1 + 1 = 2$, where "$=$" is a symbol meaning "seldom if ever"'.

Earlier in this book we learnt the beneficial features of clinical trials: there is often a control group to help put the problem in context and minor events are reported. Unfortunately, the patients in trials are not representative because, being included in the study, they are subject to protocol restraints – for example, restriction on what other medication they can take at the same time. It is sometimes the co-prescription of different medicines that causes the safety problem and such drug interactions cannot be detected in the usual clinical trial setting.

Additionally, the trialists cannot readily identify which of all the minor events they observe are caused by the drug. In fact, there is so much 'white noise' in the trial situation that, other than comparing the relative incidence of minor events in the treated group with the control group, safety information from trials is less informative than reports which are spontaneously notified to the pharmaceutical industry.

The information in 'spontaneous reports' is often presented in considerable medical detail. Additionally, the fact that the doctor has chosen to inform the company means that he or she suspects that there may be a potentially important medical issue.

Of course, if the details of the case history are inadequate this causes problems to industry and the regulators. Even so, it is important that if industry receives any information that a serious reaction is thought to have occurred it is reported to the authorities. Such information serves as an 'alert' to both industry and regulators, even if the reporter has not all the details readily at hand. However, the more complete the description and follow-up, the better the interpretation of the data and eventually, of course, the better and quicker the report of any important conclusions back to the medical profession, and the safer the medical treatment of disease.

The most florid and often the most informative sources of data are letters published in the medical journals, where both the reporter and the journal editor accept that the information may have serious clinical consequences. As published reports are important, they must be completely accurate. This is not always the case, however, as there is a temptation to 'rush into print'. It is obviously important, for example, for the hospital doctors to check their information and seek further specific details from the patient's general practitioner.

Industry also receives important information from the regulatory authorities and again this, like the spontaneous reports, is potentially medically important and suspected as being drug related – otherwise the reporting doctor would not have chosen to take the time to report it. The disadvantage of this form of reporting from industry's point of view is that for reasons of confidentiality, and quite properly, the regulatory authority is not in a position to give the pharmaceutical physicians details of the identity of the patient

and reporting doctor. Industry therefore finds it difficult or impossible to follow up many significant case histories which are initially
sent to the regulatory authority.

THE COMPANY DATABASES

Usually, within the industry, data from clinical trials are kept in a
separate database from details of spontaneous reports. Often the
serious suspected case histories from clinical trials are doubly
retained, being transferred to the database containing the spontaneous reports. This is done to focus on all serious suspected cases,
which improves the chances of finding a previously unidentified
adverse reaction to the drug.

A few years ago industry was more inclined to keep the information it received locally within its own register in that particular
country. Monitoring safety is much better with newer technology
as it is easier to fax and electronically mail safety information into
one central computerized register.

Computerization of case histories

Another advantage of the new technology is that it is easy to
itemize and produce, in a matrix, important elements from the case
histories. Examples of important parameters of information in a
group of similar cases include the time to onset of the adverse event
(in relation to start of therapy with the particular drug under
review), and whether there is a positive dechallenge or a positive
rechallenge. Listing these pieces of information helps in the
interpretation when reviewing all the data for a drug in the database.

One area of debate fascinates some workers (within the industry
and the regulatory authority) whose role it is to review large quan-
tities of data to try to identify unexpected adverse reactions, and
that is how best to handle, 'technologically', data presented as text.
For example, sclerosing peritonitis is a fibrous condition of the
peritoneum which was drug-induced by practolol (see ch. 1).
Whilst having superficial clinical similarities to adhesions following
abdominal surgery, the two conditions (sclerosing peritonitis and
abdominal adhesions), must not be combined in a computerized
database or it could possibly delay recognition of an important new
drug reaction. The original text must be preserved and the more
detailed the description of the case the easier it is to identify a

new, previously unsuspected, adverse reaction. Ideally, all fibrous peritoneal conditions should be closely related within the text-handling scheme but should also be kept distinct so that the reviewer is made aware of the more specific descriptions of the clinical events.

APPROACHES TO DATA REVIEW

Given all this important but disparate data, how does industry decide whether there is a new adverse reaction to one of its medicines?

There are two basic approaches: one is to actively and periodically review the total database looking for unusual patterns, which means that new hypotheses are being generated from within industry; the other approach, which co-exists, is to look at the relevant sections of the database when prompted by questions asked by others, to see whether their questions or hypotheses are valid. Using the first approach the reviewer does not know what he or she is seeking, but actively looks to see if there is something unusual. Using the second approach he or she is prompted to look within a certain body-system disease area of the database to see if there is supporting information for an hypothesis generated elsewhere.

Periodic database review

It is more difficult, but important, for industry to periodically review the total database, seeking any new hypotheses. By taking into account simultaneously the strength of the evidence in the individual cases (e.g. the time to onset being as expected, positive rechallenge) and the type of patient being treated (in case the apparent excess is due to the disease process rather than the drug), the aim is to identify a meaningful but new pattern of clinical events.

This approach takes discipline and is time-consuming; it requires experience and there is no mathematical way of doing it. Some companies are organized so that they are alerted automatically if, for instance, five of a particular clinical event are present, or seven. This is not totally satisfactory because, for example, seven cases of urticaria in a large database may not be very important whereas if the drug caused a serious adverse reaction, such as Stevens-Johnson syndrome, then waiting for five or seven cases could cause a significant delay.

The ad hoc review

This book is subtitled 'A Shared Responsibility' and the second, passive, approach is more likely to generate recognition of adverse reactions than the routine but disciplined review of the database, described previously, where one is not aware of what one is seeking. The passive approach relies on other people sharing the responsibility. They must continue to ask the correct questions – to generate the hypotheses to which industry responds. Those employed in drug safety units in industry are heavily dependent for hypothesis generation on questions from outside sources such as the regulators, dispensing pharmacists, the medical profession prescribing the drug and patients. It is also wise for industry to keep an eye on statements made by the manufacturers of similar drugs in case an adverse reaction to another drug in the same therapeutic class is relevant. When specific questions are asked, industry reviews the databases, writes overviews and investigates the evidence that there is a real safety issue. From what has been said previously, the clinical trial database is the best source of information for answering questions relating to type A reactions. Laboratory data is also best addressed initially in the clinical trial database. Type B reactions are usually more rare and more serious, are often specific to some patients with particular allergies, and questions relevant to type B reactions are normally best addressed by looking at spontaneous reports (including reports from the literature and reports back to industry from the regulatory authorities).

DECISION MAKING

There is no right answer when making a decision and it becomes an interesting area of medical judgement to decide whether the evidence is sufficient and the pattern clinically supportive (the time to onset is consistent etc.) for the manufacturer to decide that the time is now appropriate to alert the medical profession.

Very occasionally there is sufficient information within one well-written, fully described case history for industry doctors to choose to acknowledge the possibility of a new adverse reaction to the drug, but it is usually unwise to warn the profession when only one report exists as 'one swallow does not make a summer'. The lawyers in a company prefer any possible adverse reaction to a medicine to be immediately listed as this has an impact on product liability or compensation, but it is not helpful to the prescribing physicians if this approach is followed. It also means that for widely prescribed drugs one would reach the stage where there would be so many different single events reported, and hence the list of possibilities would be so long, that one would be tempted to say that with this drug any side-effect may happen – which is not medically helpful.

This comment is made here to indicate the sort of decisions that face both a drug safety unit in industry and the regulatory authority. It would be useful to learn the views of the practising physicians and pharmacists on these issues. The rule within a drug monitoring unit is to be alert and open-minded, actively search the database regularly, and remain aware of possible areas of importance. Higdon's law states that 'Good judgement comes from experience, experience comes from bad judgement'.

Industry's role does not stop when a comment is included in the prescribing information. There are two other issues which ought to be addressed: one is the problem of trying to identify subgroups of patients at particular risk, the other is to try and estimate the incidence or the frequency of the adverse reaction.

Identifying subgroups at particular risk

The problem with identifying subgroups of patients at particular risk is best addressed by structuring the computer output, not only so that similar case histories are aligned in close proximity, but also so that important factors, e.g. the ages of the patients and co-prescribed drugs, are listed together. As already described, some companies tend to break down the case histories into many parameters so that subgroups can be more readily identified should a problem arise. Others prefer to scrutinize the individual case reports when a new adverse reaction has been identified to see if it is possible to identify a subgroup at particular risk. If there is such a subgroup this is important not only as information for industry to pass on to the medical profession but also it can be used to suggest a pharmacological mechanism for the adverse reaction, for example the effect of renal impairment.

Estimating the frequency of the adverse reaction

Industry must also try to estimate the incidence or the frequency of a new adverse reaction and for this it must estimate how many have taken a particular medicine. Even ignoring the fact that people do not always take all the medicines that they are prescribed, and sometimes share better medicines with their friends or neighbours over their garden fence, it is difficult for industry to know how much has actually been dispensed during a given period. This is true even though it will be known how much has left the company's warehouse. This particular problem is exaggerated when reports are reviewed which originate from many different countries. Even if the manufacturers can ascertain the number of prescriptions issued, it is not possible for industry to know how many of these patients are taking the second or tenth prescription for those medi-cines used to treat chronic conditions (e.g. heart failure and arthritis) and how many prescriptions are for new patients. The numerator is also inaccurate because not all cases are notified to industry. So, once a drug is available for marketing, industry has difficulty in calculating frequency rates. This is obviously much more true for the type B reactions detectable from spontaneous reports than in clinical trials where the frequency of type A adverse reactions can be fairly accurately estimated. Having said this, industry is becoming more pro-active and tries to quote reliable incidence and frequency rates.

COMMUNICATION

De Neve's law of debate is that 'Two monologues do not make a dialogue'. One aspect of 'The Shared Responsibility' between industry doctors and those outside is that industry could better communicate the information and those outside the industry could be more pro-active in reading it! Industry is certainly trying to improve in this respect and there are initiatives to ensure that information is passed on directly from industry to the patients themselves. Information in the prescribing information in different countries worldwide is becoming more standardized, but com-placency is not in order.

What industry could possibly do better is to present the pre-scribing information on side-effects and possible adverse reactions more consistently. For example, with the passage of time a side-effect can be shown as a precaution or as a contraindication with what seems to be a small element of arbitrariness; a drug can cause bronchospasm as a side-effect and asthma may or may not be described as a precaution; some serious contraindications are shown as a warning and others are not etc.

Another problem here is not only whether a possible new adverse reaction is worthy of comment, but also which are the most appropriate words to describe the weight of the evidence. This is a matter of some concern for industry because it does not want to give information that is subsequently shown to be misleading. Often at the time that the manufacturer decides to comment in the prescribing information or data sheet, industry doctors are not certain about the relevance of the possible adverse reaction. Again, it is a matter of judgement whether one warns early, accepting that the warning may be incorrect, or whether one delays a warning until the answer is more clear-cut. Sometimes a company will deal with this situation by including a warning but wording it equivocally – however, some doctors must be irritated when the manufacturer states that there have been certain cases reported but that their interpretation or significance is not clear.

A final issue is how industry, with the regulators, can make newly identified safety issues more clearly known to the medical profession. Remember that the bottom line, our primary aim, is for the medical profession to be made more aware of safety issues so that they can more safely prescribe medicine to the patient population. One suspects that even when a serious new adverse reaction has been identified and industry sends what is called a 'Dear Doctor' letter to the prescribing physicians, or the regulatory authorities mention it in, for example, their *Current Problems* in the UK, the medical profession does not necessarily take heed of the warning. What must be done? This is a question for you, the reader, to ponder.

IN CONCLUSION

With the best will in the world, warning the medical profession about drug safety is a difficult but important task. Industry is getting better, and there is no reason to doubt that the medical profession as a whole is improving, but there is no room for complacency either inside or outside of the pharmaceutical industry. What is your role?

8. How to report suspected adverse drug reactions (ADRs)

Niall W. Balfour

INTRODUCTION

Throughout this book, the reader has been encouraged to report suspected adverse drug reactions (ADRs). All parties involved: the reporters, the patient, the pharmaceutical company and regulatory authorities benefit from this action. In chapter 4 we read that one of the 'seven deadly sins' of under-reporting of suspected ADRs was 'ignorance of how to report' (Inman 1986). This chapter aims to resolve this ignorance and highlight succinctly the mechanisms by which suspected ADRs can be reported, both to the regulatory authority and to the pharmaceutical company.

REPORTING TO THE REGULATORY AUTHORITY

The origin of ADR reporting

In 1964 Sir Derrick Dunlop, the then chairman of the Committee on Safety of Drugs (CSD), initiated a Register of Adverse Reactions. From all doctors and dentists he requested reports of 'any untoward condition in a patient which might be the result of drug treatment'. In notifying doctors and dentists he included a yellow business reply-paid postcard for the reporting of suspected reactions, and so began the UK's Yellow Card scheme for the spontaneous and voluntary reporting of suspected ADRs.

THE YELLOW CARD SCHEME

In the UK, the CSD later became the Committee on Safety of Medicines (CSM) which has a statutory duty under the Medicines Act of 1968 to promote the collection and investigation of information on ADRs. The spontaneous or voluntary reporting of ADRs by the Yellow Card scheme has had many successes, and is useful in identifying and characterizing drug hazards, identifying risk factors predisposing to ADRs, and providing some estimate of comparative toxicities within certain therapeutic groups. We have seen in chapter 4 that examples of such successes include detecting jaundice after repeated exposure to halothane and pulmonary embolism following administration of oestrogen in women of child-bearing age.

Since the scheme began the CSM has collected over 200 000 reports of suspected adverse reactions, and the annual rate of reporting has increased to almost 20 000 in 1989. The CSM is based in London but is supplemented by four regional ADR centres in Birmingham, Newcastle-upon-Tyne, Cardiff and Liverpool. The role of these regional centres is to increase ADR reporting and improve the quality of ADR reports received. They also offer a more localized information service for reporting doctors than is possible with a national body like the CSM.

Yellow Cards are readily available to the medical profession. They can be found in prescription pads, the *British National Formulary (BNF)*, the *Monthly Index of Medical Specialities (MIMS)*, the *Association of British Pharmaceutical Industries (ABPI) Data Sheet Compendium*, or they can be obtained directly from pharmacy departments of UK hospitals, from local drug information centres or by dialling 100 and asking for freephone CSM. The Yellow Card has steadily evolved through the years into its current format, as shown in Figure 8.1.

USING THE YELLOW CARD SCHEME

Currently, the CSM will only accept as valid Yellow Card reports of ADRs originating from doctors, dentists or coroners.

The reporting of ADRs associated with new drugs

When a new drug is marketed it is 'flagged' in the *BNF*, *MIMS*, the *ABPI Data Sheet Compendium* and any UK advertisement, with a black triangle ▼. This symbol is used for approximately 2 years to indicate that the safety profile of a drug is being closely monitored, particularly to identify problems not noted during clinical trials. There are special reporting requirements associated with the use of the black triangle. With these new drugs, doctors, dentists or coroners are asked to report all suspected adverse reactions,

In Confidence

COMMITTEE ON SAFETY OF MEDICINES

COMMITTEE ON DENTAL AND SURGICAL MATERIALS

REPORT ON SUSPECTED ADVERSE DRUG REACTIONS

■ **Recently introduced products**
Please report all suspected reactions, including minor ones, that could conceivably be attributed to the drug. New products are identified by a black triangle (▼) in the British National Formulary.

■ **Established products**
Please report **serious or unusual** reactions to all agents, but not minor reactions. Include reactions that are fatal, life-threatening, disabling, incapacitating, or which result in or prolong hospitalisation.

● Please also report reactions to vaccines, dental or surgical materials, IUCDs, absorbable sutures and contact lens fluids.
● Record all other drugs taken in previous 3 months including self medication.
● Report suspected drug interactions.

Do not be put off reporting because some details are not known.

REPORTING DOCTOR

Name
Address

Telephone
Speciality
Signature   Date

PATIENT'S DETAILS

Surname
Other names
Date of birth (or age)
Sex   M ☐ F ☐ Weight (kg) ☐
Hospital if relevant
Hospital number
Consultant in charge
or GP Principal

SUSPECTED DRUG

Give brand name of drug and batch number if known	Route	Daily dose	Date started	Date stopped	Therapeutic indication
			/ /	/ /	
			/ /	/ /	
			/ /	/ /	

Other drugs taken in the last 3 months including self-medication

Give brand name if known Write **None** if no other drug has been taken	Route	Daily dose	Date drug started	Date drug stopped	Therapeutic indication
			/ /	/ /	
			/ /	/ /	
			/ /	/ /	
			/ /	/ /	
			/ /	/ /	
			/ /	/ /	
			/ /	/ /	

SUSPECTED REACTIONS

	Date reaction started	Date reaction ended	Outcome eg. fatal recovered, continuing
	/ /	/ /	
	/ /	/ /	
	/ /	/ /	
	/ /	/ /	
	/ /	/ /	
	/ /	/ /	

Additional information including medical history, investigations, known allergies, suspected drug interactions relevant to the reaction and LMP for drugs taking during pregnancy.

■ If you would like information about other reports associated with the suspected drug, tick here ☐   AR 20

Fig. 8.1 The CSM Yellow Card

however minor, which could conceivably be attributed to the drug. Reports should be made despite uncertainty in the reporter's mind about a causal relationship, irrespective of whether the reaction is

Table 8.1 Guidance on examples of serious reactions to be reported to the Committee on Safety of Medicines

Blood	Cardiovascular	Central nervous system	Gastrointestinal	Immunological	Malignancy
Bone marrow dyscrasias	Arrhythmias	Anorexia nervosa	Colitis	Anaphylaxis	Any
Coagulopathies	Cardiac arrest	Cerebrovascular accident	Haemorrhage	Arteritis	
Haemolytic anaemias	Cardiac failure	Catatonia	Hepatic cirrhosis	Drug fever	
	Cardiomyopathy	Coma	Hepatic dysfunction	Graft rejection	
	Circulatory failure	Confusional state	Hepatic fibrosis	Lupus syndrome	
	Hypertension	Dependence	Ileus	Polyarteritis-nodosa	
	Hypotension	Depression	Pancreatitis	Vasculitis	
	Myocardial-ischaemia/infarction	Epilepsy (inc. exacerbations)	Perforation		
	Sudden death	Extrapyramidal reactions	Peritonitis (inc. fibrosing)		
		Hallucinations	Pseudo-obstruction		
		Hyperpyrexia			
		Intracranial hypertension			
		Myasthenia			
		Myopathies			
		Neuroleptic malignant syndrome			
		Neuropathy			
		Psychosis			
		Withdrawal syndrome			

Table 8.1 (cont.)

Metabolic	Musculoskeletal	Renal	Reproduction	Respiratory	Skin	Special senses
Acidosis	Arthropathy	Renal dysfunction	Abortion	Alveolitis (allergic, fibrosing)	Angioedema	Cataract
Adrenal dysfunction	Aseptic bone necrosis	Urinary retention	Antepartum haemorrhage	Bronchospasm (inc. exacerbation)	Bullous eruptions	Corneal opacification
Hypercalcaemia	Osteomalacia		Congenital abnormalities	Pneumonitis	Exfoliation (generalized)	Glaucoma
Hyperkalaemia	Pathological fracture		Eclampsia, pre-eclampsia	Respiratory failure	Epidermal necrolysis	Hearing loss
Hypokalaemia			Infertility	Thrombo-embolism		Vestibular dysfunction
Hyponatraemia			Uterine haemorrhage, perforation			Visual loss
Pituitary dysfunction						
Porphyria						
Thyroid dysfunction						

well recognized, and even if other drugs have been given concurrently.

The reporting of ADRs associated with established drugs

With established drugs the focus of reporting ADRs is changed. Medical professionals are no longer asked to report well described, relatively minor side-effects. However, they are asked to continue to report any event which they suspect may be an ADR and which is unusual or of a potentially serious nature. This includes reactions which are fatal, life-threatening, disabling, incapacitating or which result in or prolong hospitalization. Such events should be reported even though the adverse effect is well recognized. The CSM has issued a list of the types of serious reactions, according to therapeutic areas, of which they would always like to be made aware (Table 8.1).

The reader is reminded of when to submit a Yellow Card to the CSM in Figure 8.2.

The reporting of ADRs by pharmacists

As stated earlier, the CSM currently only accepts Yellow Card reports of ADRs from doctors, dentists or coroners. However, pharmacists, being in the unique position for drug distribution and patient liaison, could contribute greatly to the spontaneous reporting of ADRs. The Royal Pharmaceutical Society's council thus welcomed a plan for a pilot study of ADR reporting by hospital pharmacists. The 2-year study proposed by the CSM which started in January 1991 is based in the Northern Regional Drug Information Unit (Pharmaceutical Journal 1990). Pharmacists will be encouraged to complete and sign special yellow card report forms which include the name of the consultant responsible for the care of the patient as well as their own name. Within some hospitals, pharmacists can use special green cards for reporting suspected ADRs to the doctors responsible for the care of patients, so as to encourage the doctors to report via Yellow Cards. However, this scheme is not available to all UK pharmacists. This proposed pilot study of ADR reporting by pharmacists has been set up by the CSM with the aim of increasing the number of reports of suspected ADRs. As indicated in chapter 6, the subject of ADR reporting by pharmacists is controversial; however, this currently untapped and rich source of ADR information is clearly a key area for future discussion.

Should I send a Yellow Card ?

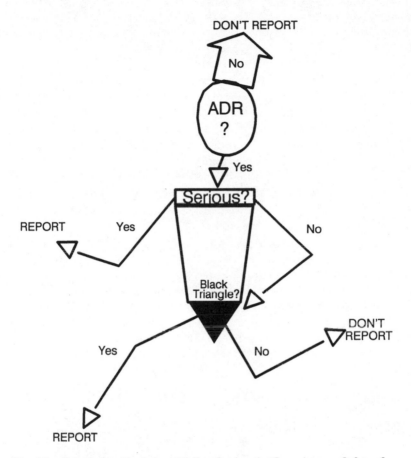

Fig. 8.2   Criteria for submitting a Yellow Card to the Committee on Safety of Medicines

Areas of special interest

The CSM have highlighted certain areas of interest which may warrant reporting in addition to the reporting requirements indicated earlier. These are:

1. Delayed drug effects – Some reactions may become manifest

months or even years after drug exposure, e.g. the 'oculo-mucocutaneous syndrome' associated with the use of practolol.

2. Drugs in the elderly – Doctors must be alert to the possibility of adverse reactions when drugs are given to the elderly, e.g. fatal liver damage mainly in elderly patients associated with the use of benoxaprofen (Opren).

3. Congenital abnormalities – When an infant is born with a congenital abnormality or when a malformed fetus is aborted, doctors are asked to consider the possibility that the malformation might be due to the effect of a drug taken by the mother during pregnancy. e.g. the use of the anticoagulant warfarin in pregnant women is associated with teratogenicity and with fetal haemorrhage near term.

4. Adverse reactions to vaccines – Vaccines are often considered in a different light from other pharmaceuticals but they too may cause adverse reactions. Since they are generally given to healthy people to reduce the risk of contracting a disease, it is most important that the risks of their use are small and very clearly defined. This becomes particularly true when, perhaps due to the vaccine's efficacy, the incidence of the disease becomes so low that the risk of damage from the vaccine exceeds that of the disease itself. It is therefore very important that adverse reactions of vaccines are reported as stringently as those occurring with drugs; e.g. polyneuritis can occur after immunization with tetanus vaccine.

Information requested by the CSM

As shown in Figure 8.1, the Yellow Card consists of six sections. Details on the following areas are requested:

1. The reporter – their name, address and telephone number, so they can be contacted should the CSM require any additional information.

2. The patient – their name, date of birth, sex, weight and hospital details, if relevant. This information will be treated in confidence.

3. The suspect drug – its trade name and batch number, if known.

4. The suspected reaction – including start and stop dates and the outcome.

5. Concurrent medication (if any).

6. Additional information.

THE REPORTING OF ADRs TO THE
PHARMACEUTICAL COMPANY BY PRESCRIBERS

The pharmaceutical company has a responsibility to monitor the safety profile of its products throughout the world and therefore needs to be informed of safety problems occurring wherever the drug is marketed. In the UK reporting of ADRs to the CSM by individual doctors is essential to raise early warning signals. However, readers are reminded that, in addition, reporting directly to the pharmaceutical company ensures that industry is alerted to a 'signal' so it can take the appropriate action, e.g. initiating data sheet changes.

Pharmaceutical companies would like to be made aware of all serious suspected ADR reports associated with their products, where 'serious' may be defined as any:

- fatal event
- life-threatening event
- event which is disabling or incapacitating
- event which required or prolonged in-patient hospitalization
- overdose, cancer or congenital anomaly
- serious laboratory abnormality associated with relevant clinical signs or symptoms.

The sooner such reports are received by the pharmaceutical company, the sooner regulatory authorities can be notified of potential problems. Pharmaceutical companies maintain a central bank of safety information on their products which include details of non-serious spontaneous reports; reporting such events is encouraged by pharmaceutical companies.

There are a number of contact points available to doctors and pharmacists for the reporting of suspected ADRs to companies. The doctor or pharmacist can contact the company's medical information department directly either by telephone or by letter. The relevant address and telephone number can be found in the *ABPI Data Sheet Compendium*, *BNF* and *MIMS*. Alternatively, doctors can contact the company indirectly by informing a visiting medical sales representative and/or providing a photocopy of the completed Yellow Card. It is then the representative's responsibility to contact the medical information department who in turn convey the message to the company's drug safety department.

Should the reader contact a pharmaceutical company to request information on a drug safety issue, the pharmaceutical company will usually attempt to determine whether the enquiry concerns a patient who has experienced an AE. When this is the case additional information will be requested by the company.

Once alerted of a suspected ADR, the company may actively follow it up, requesting relevant information. The manner of this follow-up depends on the ADR reported but in general the more serious a case, the greater is the amount of information requested. Practices vary between companies, but the doctor may be sent an adverse event form to complete if the information given initially is incomplete. Generally, company adverse event forms require information very similar to that requested on a Yellow Card. However, often they may ask for more detailed information. As was discussed in the previous chapter the data received by the company, combined with clinical trial data, will be reviewed on a regular basis to identify potential problems and implement appropriate data sheet changes. Some companies review the data so as to make a causal assessment of a case (see ch. 5). Thus, company adverse event forms may often ask for details of how a suspect ADR was treated and also the reporting doctor's assessment of causality (both in relation to the patient's original condition or other illness, and the suspect drug) so that some assessment of the drug's role in the event can be made. An example of a company's adverse event form is shown in Figure 8.3.

It is important to mention the Adverse Reaction (registration) Number issued by the CSM. If known, the reporter should include this CSM registration number on the report to the company so the company can advise the CSM and avoid duplication in their database.

WHAT THE PHARMACEUTICAL COMPANY DOES WITH THE DATA

On receipt of an ADR report, the pharmaceutical company will usually code and store the information on in-house databases in a process similar to that at the CSM. The pharmaceutical company is required by the Medicines Act of 1968 to notify the CSM of certain suspected ADRs. How the company reviews and utilizes this data together with their reporting obligations is described in detail in chapters 7 and 9.

ADVERSE EVENT REPORT FORM

CONFIDENTIAL

☒ PLEASE CROSS APPROPRIATE BOXES AND WRITE CLEARLY OR PRINT
PLEASE COMPLETE ALL SECTIONS

1. PATIENT DETAILS:
Patient identification .... Date of birth [Day] [Month] [Year]

Weight [ ] • [ ] kg   Height [ ] cms   Male ☐   Female ☐   Date of last menstrual period [Day] [Month] [Year]   Pregnant? Yes ☐ No ☐

2. RELEVANT MEDICAL HISTORY (Please include previous surgery and medical details where relevant)
....
....

3. HISTORY OF ALLERGY: (Including drug allergy)   Yes ☐   No ☐   Details: ....

4. DRUGS: (Please state suspect drug first. Include batch number where known)

		Dosage		Dates						
	Route	Unit dose	Freq.	Started			Finished			Indication
				Day	Month	Year	Day	Month	Year	

5. ADVERSE EVENT: (Please give full description, including frequency, severity, duration and diagnosis, if possible). Use additional sheet or space overleaf for Laboratory Data.

Date of onset [Day] [Month] [Year]   If time to onset is <24 hrs   Time [ ] hrs   If duration is <24 hrs   Time [ ] hrs

Description ....
....

Was the event life-threatening to this patient   Yes ☐   No ☐

6. TREATMENT OF ADVERSE EVENT:

☐ Suspect drug withdrawn due to event
☐ Dose reduced (please state new dose).............................
☐ No change in drug therapy

Did the symptoms resolve?   Yes ☐   No ☐
Was the patient rechallenged?   Yes ☐   No ☐
Did the reaction recur?   Yes ☐   No ☐

Did the event require:
Hospitalisation?   Yes ☐   No ☐
Prolongation of hospitalisation?   Yes ☐   No ☐   ← If yes, give details ....
Prescribed treatment?   Yes ☐   No ☐

7. OUTCOME:
Resolved completely ☐   Improved but still present ☐   Unchanged ☐   Worse ☐   Fatal ☐   Date [Day] [Month] [Year]

8. CAUSALITY: a. Could the **patient's original condition or other illness** account for the adverse event?
Almost certainly ☐   Probably ☐   Possibly ☐   Unlikely ☐   No ☐

b. Do you think the relationship between the **suspect drug** and the adverse event was:
Almost certain ☐   Probable ☐   Possible ☐   Unlikely ☐   Not related ☐

9. COMMENTS: (Further space on back if necessary)
....
....

10. REPORTING DOCTOR:
Name ....
Address ....
.... Tel. No.....................

11. REGULATORY AUTHORITY NOTIFIED?   Yes ☐   No ☐

12.
Date [Day] [Month] [Year]
Signature ....

Fig. 8.3 Example of an industry adverse event form

CONCLUSION

This chapter has highlighted the current system for the voluntary reporting of suspected ADRs in the UK. Effective post-marketing surveillance requires good communication and understanding between the medical profession, the MCA and the pharmaceutical company. The Yellow Card scheme may have its critics but it is currently the most effective, and certainly the cheapest, means of monitoring the safety profile of a drug. When reporting an ADR to the CSM the reporter should also consider contacting the pharmaceutical company who market the suspect drug since they too are concerned for the welfare of the patient and the safety of their drug. Pharmaceutical companies hold vast amounts of information on their products which could conceivably be of importance in future prescribing and patient management. Thus, if there is one message we would hope the reader has taken from this chapter, it is to continue and improve the shared responsibility of drug safety monitoring.

REFERENCES

Inman W H W 1986 Monitoring for drug safety, 2nd edn. MTP Press, Lancaster
The Pharmaceutical Journal 1990. Hospital pharmacists to use yellow cards in proposed CSM study. 244: 330 and 335

9. Medicines Control Agency (MCA) and other regulatory authorities

Lesley J. West

INTRODUCTION TO THE ROLE OF THE REGULATORY AUTHORITIES

Thalidomide was first marketed in Germany in 1956 for the treatment of insomnia and vomiting in early pregnancy. There was a marked increase in the incidence of congenital birth defects noted in Germany in 1961; these were typically an absence or reduction of the long bones of the limbs with normal or rudimentary hands and feet. However, the association with thalidomide was not recognized for several years after marketing with the result that thousands of babies were born worldwide with these deformities. It was evident that greater control was required to prevent such recurrences in the future.

During the mid-1960s and early 1970s several countries began to introduce legislation requiring that the safety of drugs was assessed before marketing. They also set up systems for collecting adverse drug reactions (ADRs) occurring with marketed products from both the medical profession and pharmaceutical manufacturers. This activity, stimulated by the thalidomide tragedy, was the foundation stone of safety surveillance and the start of regulatory authorities playing a significant role in ensuring drug safety. Before this some reputable companies undertook clinical trials on their new drugs but this was not legally required.

INTRODUCTION TO THE FUNCTION OF THE MEDICINES CONTROL AGENCY (MCA)

This chapter outlines the role of the MCA in the UK and in Europe, with particular respect to drug safety monitoring. The MCA functions as the drug regulatory body in the UK. Its overall function is to ensure that all medicines on the UK market meet acceptable standards of quality, safety and efficacy.

The licensing of medicines in the UK is governed by both the Medicines Act of 1968 and, since the UK is part of the European Community, the rules for medicinal products which exist in the Community. The MCA also increasingly interacts with the Committee for Proprietary Medicinal Products (CPMP) in the European Community.

It is interesting that the requirement for licensing applies not only to medicines and other therapeutic agents, but also to anything that is claimed to treat or prevent illness or to alter body function. Hence, some dental and surgical materials require a product licence. There are also anomalies and borderline cases, for example some but not all toothpastes have a product licence.

Because the regulations are written in legalistic language that can be difficult to comprehend, the MCA produces explanatory documents which set out simplified procedures for companies to apply for appropriate licences. It is the responsibility of the MCA to issue licences to those conducting clinical trials, manufacturing, exporting, importing or marketing medicinal products in the UK.

STRUCTURE OF THE MCA

Licensing of medicines in the UK is the responsibility of the Licensing Authority (Ministers) who delegate the day-to-day responsibility to officials (the MCA). The Licensing Authority is advised by a number of important advisory bodies, the most senior of which is the Medicines Commission. The Medicines Commission has responsibility, through Section 4 of the Medicines Act, to appoint additional advisory bodies, the best known of which is probably the Committee on Safety of Medicines (CSM); other Section 4 Committees are the Committee on Dental and Surgical Materials (CDSM), the Committee on Review of Medicines (CRM), the British Pharmacopoeial Commission (BPC) and the Veterinary Products Committee (VPC).

Prior to April 1st 1989, the MCA was known as the Medicines Division of the Department of Health. Following recommendations in April 1990 it was reorganized into six units each with a single 'Business Manager' who reports directly to the director (currently Dr Keith H. Jones). The Business Manager responsible for drug safety monitoring in the UK is Dr Susan Wood. Each 'Business Unit' contains a number of multi-disciplinary functional units, which are relatively small – between three to 10 staff. The structure is summarized in Figures 9.1 and 9.2.

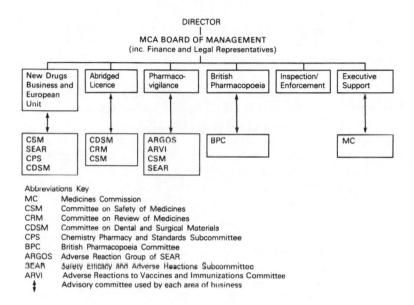

Abbreviations Key
MC   Medicines Commission
CSM   Committee on Safety of Medicines
CRM   Committee on Review of Medicines
CDSM   Committee on Dental and Surgical Materials
CPS   Chemistry Pharmacy and Standards Subcommittee
BPC   British Pharmacopoeia Committee
ARGOS   Adverse Reaction Group of SEAR
SEAR   Safety Efficacy and Adverse Reactions Subcommittee
ARVI   Adverse Reactions to Vaccines and Immunizations Committee
⥮   Advisory committee used by each area of business

Fig. 9.1   Structure of the Medicines Control Agency

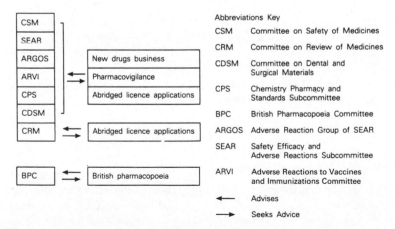

Abbreviations Key
CSM   Committee on Safety of Medicines
CRM   Committee on Review of Medicines
CDSM   Committee on Dental and Surgical Materials
CPS   Chemistry Pharmacy and Standards Subcommittee
BPC   British Pharmacopoeia Committee
ARGOS   Adverse Reaction Group of SEAR
SEAR   Safety Efficacy and Adverse Reactions Subcommittee
ARVI   Adverse Reactions to Vaccines and Immunizations Committee
←   Advises
→   Seeks Advice

Fig. 9.2   Advisory bodies to the UK Licensing System

LIFE CYCLE OF A DRUG LICENCE IN THE UK REGULATORY AUTHORITY

Clinical trial licensing before marketing

Before being administered to humans a new drug is subjected to rigorous testing in vitro and in animal studies (see ch. 2). In order to conduct clinical trials of medicinal products in the treatment of patients companies are required to obtain a clinical trial certificate (CTC) or a clinical trial exemption (CTX). The CTC is the older scheme which requires submission of comprehensive data, but is rarely used now except in special situations. The CTX requires much less data than a CTC and is now the UK standard. Well-established drugs generally need a CTX or CTC for some trials in patients, such as studies in new indications.

Applications for a CTC or a CTX are assessed by the New Drugs and European Unit. The data required from companies by the MCA for a CTX includes basic pharmaceutical data on the drug and the formulation for use. Characterization and purity of the drug substance is needed. Toxicology studies in animals must be described fully. Basic metabolic data are required and reproductive toxicity studies are needed if women of child-bearing age are included in the protocol, and mutagenicity studies are also required. Any data in volunteers must be presented. Summaries of the proposed study protocol are submitted by the company for a CTX but full details are included for a CTC.

It is possible for a CTX application to be converted into the more complex and detailed CTC if there are concerns about safety. The licence assessments are made by a Senior Medical Officer, a Principal Pharmacist and a Principal Scientific Officer. If in doubt, or if there are specific problems, the New Drugs and European Unit will seek advice from the appropriate advisory committees (see Fig. 9.2). Once a CTX or CTC has been granted, suspected ADRs reported by the company are monitored by the Clinical Trials Unit of the MCA.

Applications to market drugs

As described in Chapter 2, each regulatory authority now receives substantial evidence from animal and human studies to show whether the potential health benefit of a drug outweighs any potential side-effects before it will grant the company approval to market.

A licence is needed before medicines can be marketed but is granted only after adequate testing for quality, safety and efficacy through pre-clinical and clinical testing.

More than 90% of licence applications do not go through the advisory committees. Applications can be rejected on the grounds of safety, quality or efficacy. Companies are contacted by the MCA for specific information during the assessment of the licence. Should a licence application be refused, the company may be able to provide further information to address the concerns and the licence may be granted subsequently. A company may first appeal against a refusal to grant a licence and present their case to the CSM. In addition, second appeals can be made to the Medicines Commission (see Fig. 9.1) which is a statutory body under the Medicines Act to ensure that the Act is properly executed.

The product licences for marketed products also must be renewed at periodic intervals. Established drug substances can also form part of 'abridged' licensing procedures where, for example, approval for use of a new indication is sought, or a generic drug is to be introduced.

THE CSM AND PHARMACOVIGILANCE (THE MONITORING OF SAFETY AFTER MARKETING)

As we have seen previously, post-marketing surveillance (PMS) is important; as pre-licensing clinical trials usually include small numbers of selected patients over limited time scales, only common ADRs are generally detected in this way.

This section describes the monitoring of drug safety by the CSM after marketing. In the UK, the CSM (and CDSM) has a statutory duty under the Medicines Act of 1968 to promote the collection and study of ADR data. The Pharmacovigilance Business Unit fulfils the day-to-day responsibility of drug safety monitoring.

Pharmaceutical companies and UK regulations

In Chapter 8, we saw what information is required for completing a Yellow Card and how doctors and dentists report on Yellow Cards. This section describes the role of the pharmaceutical company in reporting ADRs. Pharmaceutical companies have a legal obligation to report suspected ADRs, unlike doctors, dentists and coroners who have no such legal obligation but are requested to report to the CSM. Reporting by pharmaceutical companies in the UK is governed by the regulations, with guidance issued by the Department of Health. Newly marketed drugs are under specific surveillance in the black triangle scheme (▼). For a description of the black triangle scheme see chapter 8. All cases of suspected reactions with 'black triangle' drugs received by companies from doctors in the UK must be reported to the CSM immediately. When the black triangle is removed only serious suspected reactions reported by UK doctors to the company need to be notified. A yellow form like the CSM Yellow Card is used to report UK cases, with additional spaces for the company name and address and product licence number. Pharmaceutical companies are also legally obliged to report foreign cases that are both serious and unexpected (not in the product data sheet).

Processing of Yellow Cards and other safety data

Inman (1986) gave the objectives of the Yellow Card scheme as follows:

1. To identify drug safety problems
2. To investigate causality
3. To facilitate benefit–risk judgements
4. To inform prescribers and patients.

On receipt of an ADR report it is given a unique identifying number and its receipt is acknowledged. The information on each Yellow Card is coded, medically assessed and then entered onto the computer. An innovative computer system has been installed called ADROIT (ADR Online Information Tracking), as described by Wood (1989). Particularly important reports may be reviewed by medical assessors and may, on occasion, require further follow-up with the reporting doctor with regional follow-up by part-time Medical Officers. In addition, reports on each 'black triangle' drug are closely scrutinized and reviewed on a monthly basis. All new reports on the system, including those from overseas, are reviewed fortnightly by a multi-disciplinary team in the MCA to check for potential safety problems. Literature is carefully monitored. The relationship between the CSM and Pharmacovigilance Business is shown in Figure 9.3 (Mann 1987).

Pharmacovigilance Business seeks advice from ARGOS for specific drug problems. This committee's only function is the review of drug safety issues, as its name suggests, 'Adverse Reaction Group Of SEAR'. ARGOS can recommend further action immedi-

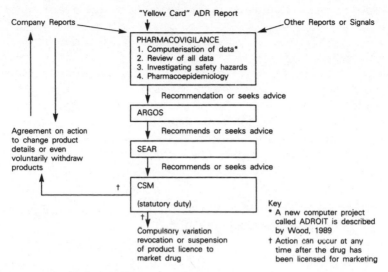

Fig. 9.3 The CSM and Pharmacovigilance

ately or refer the problem up to SEAR, the Safety, Efficacy and Adverse Reaction subcommittee of the CSM . In turn, SEAR can advise and refer a problem up to the CSM. Ultimately, the CSM may recommend the Licensing Authority i.e. responsible Government ministers to suspend and/or revoke a company product licence should the need arise.

Information provided by the MCA

As a member of the World Health Organization (WHO) Collaborating Centre for International ADR Monitoring, the MCA routinely exchanges information with WHO. The MCA also exchanges information on drug safety with other regulatory authorities. A Pharmacovigilance working group was set up in May 1989 to improve information exchange and recommend proposals for European drug surveillance. The Business also interacts with regulatory authorities outside the European Economic Community for international drug safety collaboration.

The MCA will provide computer printouts of ADR data for specific drugs on request to reporters of suspected drug reactions, including companies (West 1989, 1990). Information is always provided without revealing the identity of the doctor or patient in order to ensure confidence in the reporting system and to protect patients and doctors.

The CSM publishes *Current Problems* around four times a year to inform doctors, dentists and pharmacists of possible safety issues. Also, the 'Dear Doctor' letter is used for direct communication about particularly urgent safety issues. Journal publications and ad hoc reports may also be produced. Further details of these publications are described by Bem (1990). Lastly, Pharmaco-vigilance Business interacts with the Defect Reporting and Enforcement/inspection unit in handling clinical problems which could result from errors in manufacturing.

STANDARDIZATION OF THE ROLE OF WORLDWIDE REGULATORY AUTHORITIES

The situation for reporting post-marketing adverse events (AEs) by pharmaceutical companies is not fully standardized at present. Each authority has its own criteria for defining which events they wish to be notified about and in what time-frames. In general, regulatory authorities collect, evaluate and process all adverse reaction reports from their own countries (domestic) and selected reports from other countries (foreign). Suspected ADRs occurring in the UK will be reported by the manufacturers to some other countries (e.g. France, Germany, Italy and the USA).

Several authorities have their own regulatory forms to report events and they all record information in different formats. For example, there are CSM forms in the UK, FDA1639s in the USA and BGA forms in Germany. In addition, the FDA requires serious AEs that are not in the package insert to be reported within 15 working days, other authorities 'immediately', and yet others do not specify a time frame for reporting.

The issue of standardization has been recently addressed by a Council for International Organization of Medical Services (CIOMS) working party. It is hoped that CIOMS recommendations will become increasingly adopted by all the regulators. If regulatory authorities all agree to receive data in the same format, reporting will be more rapid, efficient and effective. There is also the added incentive to standardize within Europe in preparation for 1992, when there will be greater centralized control of the European regulators.

In some countries such as Germany and France, it is necessary for the manufacturer to submit regular detailed listings of adverse experiences in order to retain their product licence. Again, there are inconsistencies between countries in the content and format of these reports. Their standardization is the topic of a second CIOMS initiative. The plan is to include saftey updates with the regular listings.

CONCLUSION

This chapter describes the overall role of regulatory authorities with specific details about the MCA. The function and structure of the MCA are expanded with particular respect to the drug safety monitoring group.

The Yellow Card scheme is briefly outlined in terms of the Medicines Act of 1968 and the processing of those data by the MCA in the UK is explained. The obligations of pharmaceutical companies to report to the regulatory authorities both in the UK and worldwide are described.

REFERENCES

Bem J L et al 1990 25 years of the Committee on Safety of Medicines: an international perspective of the benefits. Drug Safety 5 (3): 161–167
Inman W H W 1986 Monitoring for drug safety, 2nd edn. MTP Press, Lancaster
Mann R D 1987 Adverse Drug Reactions: the scale and nature of the problem and the way forward. Proceedings of Management Forum Conference pp 5–66
West L J 1989 The ADR Section of the Medicines Control Agency. AIOPI Newsletter 6: 3–6
West L J, Thomas S, 1990 The role of the DOH Adverse Reaction Section. AIOPI Newsletter 4: 6–11
Wood S 1989 Adverse drug reactions online information tracking (ADROIT): Develoment of a new computer system to support adverse drug reaction monitoring. Pharmaceutical Medicine 4: 139–148

10. The people working in the field – careers in drug safety monitoring

Cathy J. Griffiths   Amanda J. Jukes

INTRODUCTION

Previous chapters have described various aspects of drug safety monitoring, but who are the people in this field and what do they actually do? As we have seen, drug surveillance is a relatively new but increasingly important area of health care and therefore opens up many opportunities for research physicians and scientists. Entrepreneurs are welcome! Set career paths have not been established, so this chapter aims to show the current openings and explain the daily work of some of the people in the field of drug safety monitoring.

Although the chapter concentrates mainly on drug surveillance in the pharmaceutical industry, other opportunities for careers in the health service, regulatory authorities, contract research organizations and academic centres are also addressed.

We make no apologies for describing in some detail 'life in drug surveillance' at Glaxo. We hope this will give readers a flavour of drug surveillance work in industry.

THE PHARMACEUTICAL INDUSTRY

What does industry offer?

Healthcare professionals and science graduates based in the public sector often know very little about career opportunities and working life in industry.

Pharmaceutical companies offer a wide variety of career paths for scientific personnel including biological scientists, pharmacists, physicians, statisticians, etc. Probably the most familiar figure to the outside world is the sales representative, but there are openings in basic research, pharmacy formulation, drug development, registration, information science, clinical trial design..., the list is practically endless!

Job mobility is encouraged, with scientific personnel able to move between departments in one company, and between different companies. Thus it is possible to gain a wide range of experiences to further a chosen career path.

Since much of the information required by industry about its products is found in the patient population, working in some spheres may involve local and overseas travel by the scientists and physicians who meet prescribing doctors. In a multinational company there are opportunities for even 'the backroom boys' (information scientists, systems analysts etc.) to go on overseas assignments or job secondments.

Doctors and scientists attracted into industry come from diverse career backgrounds, but all will have employed a high degree of professional integrity. In industry, maintaining this professional integrity and freedom of thought is vital to the success of the company, for example, personnel employed in drug surveillance are expected to find problems and make them known so they can be investigated, and doctors and scientists are encouraged to publish articles about their own research.

Working in drug surveillance

In previous chapters, the regulations that require pharmaceutical companies to report to regulatory authorities both individual case reports and collated safety data, were described. Because of these obligations many pharmaceutical companies have set up a central drug surveillance department to process adverse event (AE) information and fulfil reporting requirements. To achieve this effectively, it is most important that communication pathways are implemented throughout the company to ensure the fast transit of AEs to the central drug surveillance department.

Many employees in a company share this responsibility. For example, a drug representative could be told about a suspected adverse drug reaction (ADR) during a routine doctor's appointment, personnel responsible for answering product information queries may 'uncover' an AE, and of course those responsible for the conduct of clinical trials must be particularly alert to possible AEs. Because of the way that AEs are reported to the company it is imperative that the relevant employees are trained to recognize and pass on the information about AEs as quickly as possible to the central drug surveillance department.

Drug surveillance at Glaxo

At Glaxo Group Research there is an International Drug Surveillance Department (IDSD) which works to protect the health interests of the public by monitoring the safety of Glaxo products. Worldwide reports of AEs associated with Glaxo products are documented, investigated and evaluated. Reports are subsequently submitted to the appropriate worldwide regulatory authorities.

The IDSD employs healthcare professionals (e.g. physicians, epidemiologists, pharmacists, nurses), life science graduates and data specialists. This diversity of backgrounds enables the department to analyse reports from several perspectives.

Active monitoring and review of AE reports allows for the early detection of trends in safety data occurring with drugs. Post-marketing surveillance (PMS) of products allows detection of rare ADRs that may not occur during controlled clinical trials. Epidemiologic studies may be used to complement and enhance routine surveillance activity. All AE information is collated and reviewed, and numerous reports on various aspects of safety are produced (Figs. 10.1 and 10.2). Currently the department is divided into functional groups, each one responsible for an area of drug surveillance. Scientists are encouraged to rotate through the groups so they can learn all different aspects of the work, and promotion opportunities allow them to specialize in a scientific area or develop a managerial role.

Clinical trials group

AEs involving investigational drugs are reported to the 'clinical trials group'. They inform the clinical research department and investigators of any new safety issues and update the safety statements in the investigators' brochure. Regular team meetings with the clinical research department ensure that any problems with the clinical trial can be dealt with immediately. Once a study has been completed the AE profile is assessed and a safety section which discusses the laboratory data and AEs is included in the end-of-study report. This group is responsible for preparing the safety section of the registration document which is submitted to each regulatory authority to obtain a product licence.

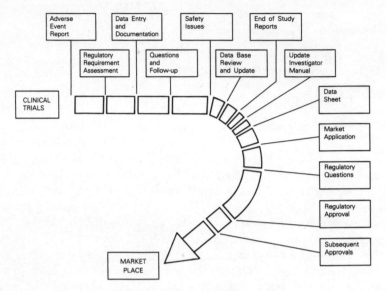

Fig. 10.1 Processing adverse event data from clinical trials

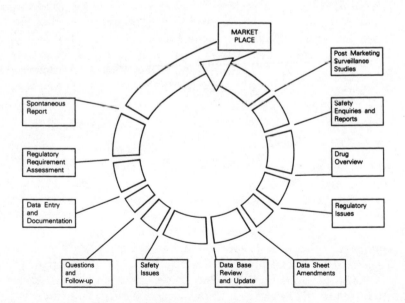

Fig. 10.2 Processing adverse event data from the marketplace

Spontaneous group

The 'spontaneous group' receives reports of marketed drugs. They write the case description and code the AEs, diseases and drugs to enable accurate searching of the database at a later date. Queries about individual cases are answered by them and they provide information regarding previous possible drug reactions to help with published cases. The group also organizes comprehensive literature searches to capture all published case reports of adverse reactions implicating Glaxo-marketed drugs. They liaise closely with local company personnel, both in the UK and overseas, in the follow-up of individual AE reports.

Drug review group

The 'drug review group' reviews all safety data on Glaxo marketed drugs. Potential new side-effects are identified and investigated to assess if they are caused by the drug. Liaison with colleagues in IDSD and other relevant departments in Glaxo is essential to complete the reviews. Safety issues are brought to the attention of the company's prescribing information safety committee which evaluates the importance of the data provided and, if necessary, recommends an update of safety statements in prescribing information documents. The drug review group also prepares answers to regulatory questions about safety, and produces routine reports to keep the regulatory authorities fully informed about the safety profile of Glaxo drugs. Reviews are stored for future reference. Protocols for PMS studies are reviewed by the group to check that relevant safety information will be collected.

Systems group

The 'systems group' works closely with all other groups in the IDSD in order to develop the most effective way of organizing the paperflow, filing, computerization and archiving of AE cases. The group manages the database and, by regulating the programming and maintaining data dictionaries, ensures that correct information is entered. This provides a source of up-to-date and accurate information of all AEs reported with Glaxo products. The database is also used to 'flag' regulatory reportable events and track their progress, thus prompting a report to be produced within the specified time-frame. Since all scientists in IDSD have to be conversant with the adverse events database and other computerized systems in the course of their work, the 'systems group' trains other members of IDSD in the use of the system. In order to offer the most effective system to the department the group must keep up to date with the latest technology and must continually improve the facility.

The role of the research physician

In IDSD the research physicians are responsible for ensuring that written material regarding drug safety is presented in an appropriate medical context. The physicians provide a medical interface between IDSD and Glaxo physicians worldwide by liaising with them in the follow-up of reported AEs and published cases. Where necessary they will visit the reporting physician to discuss the case. By attending meetings and symposia, the research physicians maintain medical contact with doctors in both the industry and the regulatory authorities, and ensure that the department is up to date with the current issues and opinions in drug surveillance worldwide. They are also responsible for initiating epidemiological studies to investigate the aetiology and progression of disease, the frequencies of illness and the factors that influence their distribution. Medical advice regarding all aspects of drug surveillance is provided by the research physicians.

Joint responsibilities

The communication of information regarding the experience of patients receiving Glaxo products is a vital function of the IDSD. Each group collaborates with other departments in Glaxo to provide medically and technically accurate responses to safety-related questions from healthcare professionals and regulatory authorities. Data may be used to aid health professionals who have encountered possible ADRs. Exchange of information between IDSD and the marketing companies and IDSD and the research departments is actively encouraged to keep the department fully informed of any issues relating to the safety of Glaxo products. This in turn enables IDSD to ensure that clinical trial investigators, prescribers of company products and patients are aware of the safety information relevant to Glaxo medicines.

In a large drug surveillance department physicians, pharmacists, pharmacologists and graduates in biological sciences all contribute to drug safety surveillance. Clinical experience, a working knowledge of hospitals, drug therapy and specialist knowledge of clinical pharmacology, pharmacokinetics, biochemistry etc., all complement each other. Although there are no officially recognized qualifications specific to drug surveillance, the Diploma of Pharmaceutical Medicine provides a background knowledge of the pharmaceutical industry for research physicians, and a number of MSc courses in clinical pharmacology are available for science graduates. Because of the diversity of drug surveillance, additional qualifications in a variety of subjects from computer sciences to management skills all improve career prospects.

Other organizations

In contrast to the drug surveillance department at Glaxo, other companies may organize their drug surveillance departments in different ways. Both the number of products marketed and type of product will influence the number of AE reports received. Commonly, AEs of pre-marketed drugs are dealt with entirely by the therapeutic division which organizes the clinical trials. In many companies, particularly subsidiaries, the responsibility of drug surveillance is only part of the role of the research scientist or physician. They may also be involved in medical affairs, marketing functions, drug information or registration. Although this often limits the scope to follow a career specifically in drug surveillance, the work is usually varied and provides experience in many different aspects of the industry in addition to safety surveillance. For some it is a good training ground before specialization.

As the quest to develop safer and more effective drugs increases, so the regulations governing the conduct of clinical trials and range of information required by regulatory authorities have grown. A pharmaceutical company may have several drugs in the investigational phase and demands upon staff may fluctuate depending upon the success and progress of each new drug. This situation has led to the development of contract research organisations which will take over all or some of the investigational stage of new drugs, including the management of safety data. They offer experience with a range of drugs from different companies.

REGULATORY AUTHORITIES

Opportunities for careers in drug surveillance exist in regulatory authorities which employ scientists and physicians to assess the safety of drugs prior to their acceptance onto the market, and subsequently. Physicians assess the data provided by pharmaceutical companies before a licence can be granted for a drug to go into the development phase of clinical trials, and again when the final product licence application is submitted. Pharmacists assess the formulation, pharmacokinetics and pharmacodynamics of the drug. Yellow Cards are collected and the information documented in a computer system by scientists for future reference. Scientists may also work in specialist roles according to their qualifications. The regulatory authority assesses the suspected ADRs received and has the right to investigate the company and, if necessary, authorize the drug to be withdrawn from the market. Information is also distributed to doctors and pharmacists to warn of the current problems associated with particular drugs (see ch. 9).

The World Health Organization is an extension of the individual countries' regulatory authorities and maintains a worldwide database of suspected ADRs. With the advent of the European Common Market a European Pharmacovigilance Centre will be set up and have a similar role. Much work is underway at the moment to rationalize the functions of the various regulatory authorities.

THE HEALTH SERVICE

In the Health Service prescribing doctors have the main responsibility for drug safety through safe prescribing. However, with the development of newer and more potent drugs, and their success in the treatment of diseases which previously did not respond to medication, the number of drugs prescribed and the treatment period for each patient has increased. Unfortunately, the risk of developing side-effects has also increased as a consequence; however, various measures have been introduced to facilitate the safe prescribing of drugs.

Hospitals have direct access to drug information centres which are usually run by pharmacists, and regional reporting centres which receive Yellow Cards directly, have been set up in four hospitals. These centres were set up initially both to increase doctors' awareness of the importance of reporting AEs, and also to collect follow-up information, where possible, to improve the quality of reports which are then sent on to the Committee on Safety of Medicines (CSM).

Pharmacists have a particularly important role in drug safety. In hospitals they monitor prescriptions on the wards for each patient and may advise the prescribing doctor of any potential drug interactions, inappropriate dose regimens or possible side-effects associated with the drugs. They may recommend therapeutic drug monitoring and discuss how the patient's disease can influence the drug metabolism and action, and identify any associated changes in biochemistry parameters that the drug may cause. Pharmacists are also responsible for ensuring that drugs are prescribed at the recommended doses.

FURTHER CAREER OPTIONS

As worldwide awareness of the importance of drug safety has increased so has the importance of epidemiological studies and the necessity to find out how drugs on the market affect the patient. This has led commercial companies to set up computerized record linkage systems. These systems track patient records retrospectively and prospectively and link the drug, the patient's medical history, concurrent illness and drug therapy together. They enable disease patterns and AEs to be studied in various patient populations. This is particularly useful in PMS (see ch. 3). These commercial companies provide another potential route for physicians and scientists to develop careers in drug safety.

Several academic centres are closely involved in drug safety. At Southampton University a department is funded to improve the safety of marketed drugs through prescription event monitoring (PEM) (see ch. 3). Formal centres have not been set up to evaluate and investigate methods of drug surveillance; however, links have been established between academic centres, hospitals, regional reporting centres and the regulatory authorities by individuals who work there. This encourages exchange of information regarding drug surveillance.

There are a number of associations which doctors, pharmacists and scientists may join to keep abreast of safety issues. We have included a few here for your reference; however, this list is by no means complete.

ACRPI – Association of Clinical Research in the Pharmaceutical Industry

BAPP – British Association of Pharmaceutical Physicians

BIRA – British Institute of Regulatory Affairs
DIA – Drug Information Association
ISPE – International Society of Pharmacoepidemiology

We hope this chapter has given you a taste of what some of the people do who work in the world of drug surveillance. Has it whetted your appetite to join them?

11. Information sources

John C.C. Talbot   Lesley J. West

INTRODUCTION

A common clinical problem facing doctors is 'has the patient experienced an adverse drug reaction (ADR)?' In addition to evaluating the merits of each individual case, i.e. timing, presentation, dechallenge etc., the question is 'has this ADR been reported with the drug before?' This chapter briefly reviews what information sources are available to provide the answer. The first part of the chapter considers the value of individual published case reports and what information these should include; it goes on to consider briefly literature-searching and the secondary information sources that are available. The second part is a bibliography listing the key books and other information sources with pointers to their use and value.

PUBLISHED LITERATURE

The publication of individual case reports in medical or scientific journals is a key primary source of information on ADRs. Unlike reports received by regulatory authorities or by the pharmaceutical industry, the details of published cases are available to all. Published reports are also seen to have a high degree of credibility and are cited by other authors despite the uncertainty of a cause–effect relationship in many cases. The quality of reports in the literature is extremely variable and has been the subject of much criticism and debate. In response to this, minimum information elements for reports have been proposed (Jones 1982) and some journals issue guidelines or checklists for prospective authors (Anon 1991). Table 11.1 presents a suggested list of what should be included in an ADR case report.

Journals should publish reports of suspected ADRs although

Table 11.1   What information should be included in an adverse drug reaction (ADR) report?

Item	Details
Patient details	Age, sex, body-weight, race
Medical history	Relevant history and concurrent conditions, environmental factors, prior experience with drug, ADRs with similar drugs
Timing	How long had the patient been receiving the drug before the suspected ADR? Details of other drugs, dose, duration, indication etc.
Dechallenge	Was the suspect drug stopped? Were other drugs stopped? What was the outcome and what was the time course?
Alternative causes	What other conditions or factors could have accounted for the ADR, which ones were excluded?
Rechallenge	Was the patient rechallenged? What was the effect, time course etc?
Verifying factors	Blood levels, laboratory data, biopsy findings
Other reports	Literature, regulatory authority, pharmaceutical company

there is always the risk of false alarms. Editors should aim to steer a path between the extremes of 'crying wolf' too often and insisting on near certain evidence. They should also ensure that the quality of the case reports is high. Unfortunately, there is often a surprisingly long delay between the occurrence of a suspected ADR and its appearance in the published literature. Haramburu et al (1985) found a mean delay of 69 weeks, which emphasizes the importance of notifying the regulatory authority and pharmaceutical company at the time the ADR occurred. Pharmaceutical companies are also required to report certain published cases and pre-publication manuscripts to the regulatory authorities.

Searching the literature

In the ever-increasing number of biomedical journals there are frequent reports of suspected ADRs. For older drugs these may go back many years and are best located using secondary information sources. However, for newer drugs first reports may have only recently been published, and not necessarily in a UK journal or an English language journal, such is the international nature of the subject. 'On-line' literature searching of commercial databases such as MEDLINE (Index Medicus), EMBASE (Excerpta Medica) and RINGDOC has become available to more and more users in recent years. These databases partly overcome the lag-time a paper takes to be included in reference books but it still takes a while for a paper to be indexed and entered onto the database. They are also not entirely comprehensive in journal coverage, particularly for conference abstracts and proceedings. Indexers who compile the entries also apply certain selection criteria to restrict the number of index terms used, which may result in some drugs or ADRs being missed if they are a secondary part of the paper. There is also the problem of 'false drops'. If a search is conducted using the appropriate terms for a drug and an ADR a list of references indexed with these terms will be obtained. However, the papers retrieved do not necessarily describe a case in which the drug causes the ADR because it is not usually possible to link the index terms for the drug and ADR directly. Reference to the drug being used in the treatment of a patient with that disease or reaction and separate coincidental mentions may also be selected.

Secondary information sources

Secondary information sources use the primary publications described previously. They include abstracts, reviews, the Committee on Safety of Medicines (CSM) publication *Current Problems* and finally reference books about ADRs. There are a number of excellent reference books on ADRs, the 'gold standard' being *Meyler's Side-effects of Drugs* and *Meyler's Side-effects of Drugs Annuals*. However, the problem with all such reference books is the delay between a suspected ADR being reported in the literature and its inclusion in the publication. This is a particular problem with new drugs and newly reported ADRs with more established drugs. The delay between a reaction becoming well-established in the published literature and appearing in *Current Problems* was shown to be between 0 and 5 years (Twomey & Griffin 1983).

Meyler's *Side-effects of Drugs* is now available 'on-line' as SEDBASE, overcoming the delay in publication to an extent, although, only certain categories of drugs are incorporated. The ADR-specific publication *Reactions* published by ADIS Press, New Zealand, provides brief abstracts on important ADRs appearing in the literature and has a lag-time of only a few weeks. In 1990 it became a weekly rather than biweekly publication and is now known as *Reactions Weekly*. There is also a similar US publication called *Clin-Alert*. Drug information pharmacists in the UK also run a database called Pharmline. This includes papers on all aspects of drug therapy but about a quarter concern ADRs. It is available on DATASTAR and provides a useful and relatively cheap source of information.

SELECTED SOURCES OF INFORMATION ON SPECIFIC ADR TOPICS

Sources of information are diverse. Many publications and on-line services contain reports and reviews about ADRs and related topics, as described previously. No attempt is made here to cover the whole range of sources. The following lists indicate selected publications and on-line information relating to particular ADR topics.

1.   Post-marketing ADR monitoring

Specific books on drug surveillance

1.1   *Monitoring for Drug Safety* edited by W H Inman with assistant editor E P Gill. Published by MTP Press Limited, a member of the Kluwer Academic Publishers Group. The second edition was published in 1986 (ISBN 0 85200 721 3).

1.2   *Adverse Drug Reactions. The Scale and Nature of the Problem and the Way Forward*, edited by R D Mann. Published by Parthenon Publishing Group in 1987 as proceedings of a conference organized by Management Forum Ltd (ISBN 1 85070 137 7 and 0 940813 13 0). Updates of chapters by R D Mann are published in *Risk and Consent to Risk in Medicine*, proceedings of a conference by Management Forum Ltd in 1988 (ISBN 1 85070 263 2).

1.3   *Monitoring for Adverse Drug Reactions* edited by S R Walker and A Goldberg. Published in 1983 by MTP Press Limited, a member of the Kluwer Academic Publishers Group, as proceedings of the Centre for Medicines Research Workshop held at the Ciba Foundation in London (ISBN 0 85200 876 7).

1.4   *The Detection of New Adverse Drug Reactions*, by M D B Stephens. The second edition was published by Macmillan in 1988. Also covers pre-marketing, regulations and data management (ISBN 0 333 45417 0).

Specific journals on drug surveillance

1.5   *Reactions Weekly. Alerts to Adverse Drug Experience* is published weekly, 50 times a year with monthly, 6-monthly and annual cumulated indexes (ISSN 0157 7271). It is published by ADIS Press and now available on-line via IMSBASE.

1.6   *Adverse Drug Reaction Bulletin* published every 2 months by Meditext (ISSN 0044 6394), edited by D M Davies. Also originating from Meditext and then published every quarter by Oxford University Press is *Adverse Drug Reactions and Acute Poisoning Reviews* (ISSN 0260 647X).

1.7   *Clin-Alert* is published semi-monthly by Clin Alert Inc. It contains monographs on publications relevant to exceptional situations encountered in the use of modern therapeutic agents and procedures (ISSN 0069 4770).

1.8   *Drug Information Journal* is the official publication of the Drug Information Association in the USA and members receive the journal as part of their annual subscription. It is published quarterly by Pergamon Journals Ltd (ISSN 0092 8615).

1.9   *Current Problems* is published by the CSM three to four times a year, or when necessary. *Current Problems* seeks to describe newly recognized ADRs and to advise on ADR reporting.

1.10   *Drug and Therapeutics Bulletin,* published fortnightly by Consumers' Association Ltd 1991, includes ADR information. There are cumulative indexes.

2.   Prescribing and other sources containing ADR information

2.1   *ABPI Data Sheet Compendium,* published every year by Datapharm Publications Ltd of 12 Whitehall, London SW1A 2DY. Available automatically and free of charge to physicians in the UK. Other copies available from Datapharm on 071 930 3477 (ISBN 0 907102 04 2). Note that abbreviated data sheet information is available in electronic form (PHILEX from Exeter Database Systems Ltd). Data can be displayed but not searched using a microcomputer, or is available via Meditel's ABIES.

2.2   *British National Formulary (BNF),* published about twice-yearly by the British Medical Association and the Pharmaceutical Society of Great Britain has abbreviated information on ADR and drug interactions (ISBN 0 85369 251 3). Similarly, *MIMS Monthly Index of Medical Specialities* published by MIMS also contains brief information.

2.3 *Martindale. The Extra Pharmacopoeia*, edited by J E F Reynolds. Published by The Pharmaceutical Press. The first edition was published in 1883 and the current 29th edition in 1989 (ISBN 0 85369 210 6). *Martindale* is also available on-line via Data-Star or Dialog.

3. Books and journals relating to drug interactions

Drug interaction journals

3.1 *Drug Interactions Newsletter. A Clinical Perspective and analysis of Current Developments* is published monthly by Applied Therapeutics Inc. and edited by P D Hansten and J R Horn. It contains monographs on drug interactions and *Updates of Moderate or Major Clinical significance* (ISSN 0271 8707).

Specific books on drug interactions

3.2 *Drug Interactions. A Source Book of Adverse Interactions, their Mechanisms, Clinical Importance and management*, edited by I Stockley. Published in 1981 by Blackwell Scientific Publications (ISBN 0 632 008431).

3.3 *A Manual of Adverse Drug Interactions* edited by J P Griffin, P F D'Arcy and C J Spiers. The fourth edition was published in 1988 (ISBN 07236 05440) by Wright.

3.4 *Drug Interactions*, by P D Hansten and J R Horn 6th edition 1989. This is an essential reference text, arranged in broad drug groups with an alphabetical drug interaction index (ISBN 0 8121 123 2, in loose leaf folder).

3.5 *Clinical Pharmacology of Drug Interactions*, edited by R Rondanelli. Published by Piccin in 1988 (ISBN 0 88416 034 3). Covers general considerations, then specific drugs or drug group interactions.

Sources containing relevant information on drug interactions

3.6 *Iatrogenic Disease*, edited by P F D'Arcy and J P Griffin (ISBN 0 19 261440 1), chapter 39. Also, *Textbook of Adverse Drug Reactions* edited by D M Davies (ISBN 0 19 261479 7), appendix 1. Both books are published by Oxford University Press. The third editions came out in 1986 and 1985 respectively.

3.7 INTERLEX is a pc-based information system on drug interactions, obtained from Exeter Data Base systems Ltd. It is edited by Dr L Beeley and is updated approximately every 6 months. Drug interaction in the BNF and INTERLEX are similar.

4. Teratogenicity

Specific books on drug-induced teratogenicity

4.1 *Birth Defects and Drugs in Pregnancy*, edited by O P Heinonen, D Slone and S Shapiro. Published by Publishing Sciences Group, Inc., in 1977 (ISBN 0 88416 034 3).
4.2 *Clinical Aspects of the Teratogenicity of Drugs*, by H Nishimura and T Tanimura. Published by Excerpta Medica and American Elsevier Publishing company Inc. in 1976 (ISBN 90 21920934).
4.3 *Drugs as Teratogens*, edited by J L Schardein. Published in 1976 by CRC Press Inc. (ISBN 0 87819 099 6).

5. Drug effects on lactation

Specific books on drugs and human lactation

5.1 *Drugs and Human Lactation*, edited by P N Bennett. Published by Elsevier in 1989 (ISBN 0 444 90361 5[US]). Co-editors and members of the WHO working group contributed to this useful book. Epidemiology, pharmacokinetics and effects of specific drug or drug groups are covered.

Sources containing relevant information on drug use during breast feeding

5.2 *Textbook of Adverse Drug Reactions* edited by D M Davies (ISBN 0 19 261479 7). Information included in chapter 6 of the third edition, published in 1985 by Oxford University Press.
5.3 There are various classification systems for drug use during breast-feeding (and pregnancy). One example is *Acta Obstetricia et Gynecologica Scandinavica* 1984 Supplement 126 'Drug use during pregnancy and breast-feeding: a classification system for drug information' (ISBN 0300 8835).

6. Excipients

6.1   *Textbook of Adverse Drug Reactions*, edited by D M Davies, third edition 1985 (ISBN 0 19 261479 7), appendix 2 'Adverse reactions attributed to pharmaceutical excipients'. Published by Oxford University Press.

6.2   *Excipients: Handbook of Pharmaceutical Excipients* published by the American Pharmaceutical Association and The Pharmaceutical Society of Great Britain in 1986 (ISBN 0 85369 164 9).

6.3   *Formulation factors in adverse reactions.* First of a 'Topics in Pharmacy Services' by A T Florence and E G Salole, published by Wright, 1990 (ISBN 0 7236 0923 3).

6.4   A two part authoritative review is published in *Medical Toxicology* 1988:3:128–65 and 209–40, by Larry K Golightly et al.

6.5   Specific *Current Problem* articles by the CSM are concerned with adverse reactions to excipients and found in *Current Problems* issue numbers 10, 13, 15, 22 and 23.

7. General

7.1   *Meyler's Side-effects of Drugs*, edited by M N G Dukes, eleventh edition 1988 (ISBN 0 444 90484 0). Expensive, but the definitive reference work.

7.2   *Meyler's Side-effects of Drugs Annuals*, edited by M N G Dukes, Annual 14 published 1990.

REFERENCES

Anon 1991 Guidelines for writing papers. Adverse drug reactions checklist. British Medical Journal 302: 40–42

Haramburu F, Begaud B, Pere J C, Marcel S, Albin H 1985 Role of medical journals in adverse drug reaction alerts. Lancet ii: 550–551

Jones J K 1982 Criteria for journal reports of suspected adverse drug reactions. Clinical Pharmacy 1: 554–555

Twomey C E J, Griffin J P 1983 The information lag – has it improved? Pharmacy International 4: 57–61

Glossary

Neelam Patel   Lewit A. Worrell

ABPI, The Association of the British Pharmaceutical Industry. Trade association of the UK pharmaceutical industry which acts as a channel of communication and assists contact between member companies and government departments, professional bodies etc. It represents industry in matters with the UK government regarding pricing of drugs, has a code of practice committee and produces the data sheet compendium etc.

ADR, adverse drug reaction (*see* Adverse reaction).

Adverse reaction. 'Any response to a drug that is noxious and unintended and that occurs at doses used in man for prophylaxis, diagnosis, or therapy, excluding failure to accomplish the intended purpose' (Karch & Lasagna 1975, ch. 1). Note that it is considered that an adverse reaction is causally related to the drug.

AE, ADE, adverse event. 'A particular untoward happening experienced by the patient undesirable either generally or in the context of his disease' (Finney 1965, ch. 1). Note that the adverse event may or may not be causally related to the drug.

Algorithm. A step-by-step method for solving a problem; a decision tree.

ARGOS, Adverse Reaction Group of SEAR. A subcommittee of the Committee on Safety of Medicines with specific interest in drug surveillance.

BARDI, Bayesian Adverse Reaction Diagnostic Instrument. A method for the assessment of the causality of an adverse event.

Benefit. The therapeutic efficacy of a drug.

BGA, Bundesgesundheitsamt. Authority controlling the safety and use of medicines within Germany.

Black triangle (▼). A symbol used by the Committee on Safety of Medicines to 'flag' prescribing information on all new drugs marketed in the UK; it indicates that suspected adverse drug reactions associated with that drug must be closely monitored and reported to the Committee.

BNF, British National Formulary. A publication of the British Medical Association and the Royal Pharmaceutical Society of Great Britain. Contents include UK guidance on prescribing, classified notes on drugs and preparations, dental practitioner's formulary and Yellow Cards for reporting reactions.

Case-control study. Epidemiological investigation in which subjects with a disease are compared to subjects without the disease with regard to a previous exposure to certain risk factors. (e.g. a particular drug).

CIOMS, Council for the International Organization of Medical Sciences. International non-governmental organization interested in standardizing adverse event reporting worldwide. It operates under the auspices of the World Health Organization.

Cohort study. Epidemiological investigation in which one group of subjects exposed to a risk factor (e.g. a drug) and, usually, another group not exposed to that risk factor, are followed up and compared with regard to emergent patterns of disease.

CSD, Committee on Safety of Drugs. A group formed prior to the Committee on Safety of Medicines that was involved in the approval and safety monitoring of medicines.

CSM, Committee on Safety of Medicines. An expert committee (appointed by Ministers) that advises the Licensing Authority on safety, quality and efficacy of new medicines for human use and monitors adverse reactions to medicines already on the market.

CPMP, Committee for Proprietary Medicinal Products. A representative group dedicated to the licensing of medicines in Europe.

CTC, clinical trial certificate. The older of two licences granted by the Licensing Authority in the UK to permit the administration of new chemical entities to patients. To secure such a licence involves the submission of comprehensive exploratory data (*see* CTX).

CTX, clinical trial exemption. A licence granted by the Licensing Authority for a clinical trial of a new medicine in the UK. It is the more commonly employed licence used by pharmaceutical companies.

Data sheet. Company document which contains basic information about the composition, uses, dosage, side-effects, contraindications and warnings relating to a medicine.

Dechallenge. The withdrawal of a drug after a possible adverse reaction has occurred. The response to dechallenge is a major factor used in the assessment of drug causality (see ch. 5).

Epidemiology. The study of the distribution and determinants of disease frequency in the population.

FDA, Food and Drug Administration. Authority which monitors the use of medicines and foods (including cosmetics and medical devices) within the USA.

Global introspection. An unstructured mental process whereby the facts concerning a patient and their disease are integrated to form a diagnosis.

Indication. Any disease, illness, sign or symptom presented by a patient, to which a drug treatment is targeted.

Investigator. Medical doctor involved in the running of a clinical trial.

Investigator's brochure. Company document given to an investigator to enable him to conduct a safe and ethical clinical trial. This document summarizes information on drug chemistry, toxicology, use in man, clinical safety etc.

Medicines Commission. The only statutory body under the Medicines Act, charged with the responsibility of seeing that the Act is properly executed. A function of the Commission is to hear appeals against Committee on Safety of Medicines decisions.

MCA, Medicines Control Agency. The regulatory authority in the UK, part of the Department of Health, concerned with licensing of medicines and monitoring safety.

Medicines Act 1968. Comprehensive legal framework of control in which the licensing of medicines should be procured and maintained.

NCE, New chemical entity. Term used to describe any new drug in development.

PEM, Prescription event monitoring. An initiative pioneered by Professor W Inman at the Drug Safety Research Unit, depending on information obtained from the Prescription Pricing Authority which enables adverse event monitoring of patients receiving pre-selected drugs in general practice.

Pharmacodynamics. The study of the mechanism of action of drugs and their effects on the physiology and biochemistry of the human body.

Pharmacoepidemiology. Application of epidemiological techniques to the study of drugs, especially drug safety.

Pharmacokinetics. The study of the absorption, distribution, biotransformation and excretion of drugs. These factors, coupled with dosage, determine the concentration of drug at sites of action.

Phase I. First introduction of a new drug into man (often healthy volunteers). Its main purpose is to identify dose-related adverse drug reactions and to provide a first outline of the pharmacokinetic/dynamic profile.

Phase II. Second phase of clinical drug development performed in selected populations of patients, the purpose of which is to gather efficacy and safety data specific to an indication or disease, and also to establish dosages to be employed in phase III.

Phase III. Close monitoring of drug efficacy and drug safety, in patients for whom the drug is intended, prior to market approval. All adverse events are closely monitored, with the emphasis placed on severity, duration, etc.

Phase IV. Targeted clinical studies conducted after marketing of the medicinal product.

Placebo. A pharmacologically inactive substance administered in a clinical trial.

PMS, post-marketing surveillance. Systematic process of monitoring the safety of marketed drugs to identify new 'signals', or to test hypotheses.

Pre-marketing clinical trials. Clinical trials designed to signal efficacy, safety etc. of a new drug. Generally considered to comprise phases I, II and III (see above).

Product liability. This is the concept addressing the question of who has responsibility and what redress is available when a patient suffers injury as a result of taking a medicinal product.

Rechallenge. The deliberate or inadvertent administration of a further dose(s) of the same drug to a person who had previously experienced an adverse event, which might be drug-related. The response to rechallenge is a major factor used in the assessment of drug causality (see ch. 5).

Record linkage. Bringing together of data on the same individuals, from different sources, e.g. linking hospital discharge data with patients' general practitioner prescriptions.

Risk. The liability of a drug to cause side-effects.

Safety profile. History of a drug's safety record.

SEAR, Subcommittee on Safety, Efficacy and Adverse Reactions. Subcommittee of the Committee on Safety of Medicines involved with drug safety surveillance and evaluation of new drugs.

Side-effect. A non-specific term used in this book to describe an unwanted effect of a drug but not discriminating between an adverse reaction and an adverse event. Note the term is sometimes used to imply an adverse reaction predictable on pharmacological grounds.

Spontaneous reporting. Voluntary reporting of adverse events to regulatory authorities, pharmaceutical companies or journals; reports may be received from health professionals, consumers, lawyers, etc. This form of reporting may signal the occurrence of previously undetected adverse reactions.

Strict liability. An aspect of recent UK law which makes the manufacturer liable if a medicine is defective, i.e. it causes an adverse reaction which was not identified and notified to the prescriber prior to the time of prescribing. Negligence does not have to be proven, only that injury has taken place.

Type A reaction. An augmented pharmacologically predictable reaction which is dose-dependent. It is generally associated with a high morbidity and low mortality.

Type B reaction. A bizarre reaction which is unpredictable pharmacologically and is independent of dose. It is generally associated with a low morbidity and high mortality.

WHO, World Health Organization. Organization established to promote global health and wellbeing.

Yellow Card scheme. Existing scheme for spontaneous reporting of UK adverse reactions by doctors, dentists, coroners, medical authors and the industry to the Committee on Safety of Medicines.

Index

ABPI *see* Association of the British
Pharmaceutical Industry
ADE *see* Adverse event
ADR *see* Adverse drug reactions
ADROIT *see* Adverse Drug Reaction
Online Information Tracking
Adverse drug reaction, 3, 37, 117
characterization, 40, 44, 72–73
detection, 48–52
dose-dependent, 41
follow-up of, 86
hypothesis, 36
identification, 41, 60
in elderly, 84
known, 51
management of, 60
mechanism, 48, 73
monitoring, 112
numbers required to detect, 21
profile, 27
Type A, 4, 17, 18, 19, 20, 39, 48, 72,
121
Type B, 4, 20, 48, 72, 122
see also Hypothesis generation;
Incidence rates; Reporting
Adverse Drug Reaction Online
Information Tracking, 94
AE *see* Adverse event
Adverse event, 3, 23, 29, 117
data processing, 101–103
forms, 39, 48, 54, 87
Adverse reaction *see* Adverse drug
reaction
Adverse Reaction Group of SEAR, 94,
117
Adverse reaction profile *see* Adverse
drug reaction, profile
Algorithm, 52, 117
Ames test *see* Toxicological evaluation,
Ames test
Anaphylaxis, 39

Animal studies, 92
Animal toxicity, 14
ARGOS *see* Adverse Reaction Group
of SEAR
Association of the British
Pharmaceutical Industry, 5, 32,
78, 117

BARDI *see* Bayesian Adverse Reaction
Diagnostic Instrument
Bayesian Adverse Reaction Diagnostic
Instrument, 53–54, 117
Bayes' theorem, 53
Benefit–risk, 58
assessment, 14
ratio, 1
Black triangle, 34, 78, 94, 118
BNF *see* British National Formulary
Boston Collaborative Drug Safety
Programme, 35
British National Formulary, 78, 118

Carcinogenicity *see* Toxicological
evaluation, carcinogenicity
Careers in drug safety, 99–108
Case-control studies *see*
Epidemiological studies, case-
control studies
Case reports 37, 38
publication, 58, 69, 103, 109
quality, 39
Causal relationship, 4, 24, 40, 86
assessment of, 47–56
methods, 52–55
CIOMS *see* Council for the
International Organization of
Medical Sciences
Class statements, 10
Clinical investigator's brochure *see*
Investigator's brochure
Clinical record form, 22, 23

Clinical signs and symptoms, 22
Clinical trial certificate, 92, 118
Clinical trial exemption, 92, 118
Clinical trials, 2, 13–26
  controlled, 2
  multicentre, 22
  multiple dose, 18
  phase I, 16–19, 120
    aims, 17
    methods, 17–18
  phase II, 19–25, 120
  phase III, 19–25, 120
  phase IV, 27, 120
  pre-marketing, 9, 120
  single dose, 17, 18
  see also Epidemiological studies
Cohort Studies see Epidemiological
  studies, cohort
Committee for Proprietary Medicinal
  Products, 90, 118
Committee on Safety of Drugs, 77, 118
Committee on Safety of Medicines, 32,
  34, 37, 58, 77, 90, 93, 107, 118
  Pharmacovigilance Business Unit, 93
Compensation, 67, 73
Confidentiality, 60, 61
Congenital abnormalities, 84
Contract research organizations, 105
Co-prescription, 69
Council for the International
  Organization of Medical
  Sciences, 96, 118
CPMP see Committee for Proprietary
  Medicinal Products
CSD see Committee on Safety of Drugs
CSM see Committee on Safety of
  Medicines
'Current Problems', 75, 96, 111

Database, 37, 44–45, 70–72, 86, 103
  original text preservation, 70
  review, 71
Data review, 71–72
Data sheet, 4, 21, 25, 55, 74–75, 119
DATASTAR, 112
'Dear Doctor' letter, 9, 75, 96
Dechallenge, 49, 50, 70, 119
Delayed drug effects see Latent period
Department of Health, 90
Dictionaries, coding, 103
Differential diagnosis, 49–52
Doctor–patient relationship, 64
Drug causality see Causal relationship
Drug development, 13
Drug-induced effect, 47
Drug interaction, 51, 114

Drug representative see Medical sales
  representative
Drug surveillance department, 48, 100
Drug surveillance journals, 113
Duration of exposure, 14

EMBASE, 110
End-of-study report, 101
Epidemiological studies, 28–31, 104,
  107
  case-control, 30–31, 35, 40, 118
  cohort, 29–30, 35, 40, 118
European community, 90, 95
Exclusion criteria, 2

Global introspection, 52, 119
'Green form', 34

Health care professional
  career, 106
  interface with industry, 57–65
  investigator, 119
  role in surveillance, 8–9
  role of investigator, 22
Health cooperatives, 36
Hypothesis generation, 40, 44, 71
  in industry, 72
  outside industry, 72

Iatrogenic disease, 7, 114
IMS see Intercontinental Medical
  Statistics
Incidence rates, 6, 41, 73, 74
  type A reactions, 74
  type B reactions, 21, 74
Industry, role of see Pharmaceutical
  industry, role of
Information sources, 109–116
Interaction see Drug interaction
Intercontinental Medical Statistics, 40
Investigator see Health care
  professional, investigator
Investigator's brochure, 9, 24, 101, 119

Laboratory tests, 22, 51
Latent period, 39, 83–84
LD_{50} see Toxicological evaluation, LD_{50}
Liability, 59, 61, 73, 121
Litigation, 7
Longterm safety, 2

Marketing department, 60
Marketing licence, 27
  see also Product licence application
MCA see Medicines Control Agency
Medical department, 60, 85

Medical sales representative, 85, 99, 100
Medicines Act 1968, 5, 77, 86, 90, 119
Medicines Commission, 90, 93
Medicines Control Agency, 89–97, 119
    advisory committees, 91
    Clinical Trials Unit, 92
    function, 89–90
    New Drugs Unit, 92
    structure, 90–91
Medicines (Data Sheet) Regulations 1972, 5
Medicines Division, 90
MEDLINE, 110
MEMO, 35
Meyler's Side-effects of Drugs, 111
MIMS see Monthly Index of Medical Specialities
Monthly Index of Medical Specialities, 47, 78

National Health Service, 34
NCE see New chemical entity
Negligence, 59
New chemical entity, 120

Oculomucocutaneous syndrome, 3
    with practolol, 3

Package leaflet see Patient guidance leaflet
PACT see Prescribing Analysis and Costs
Patient, 7
Patient guidance leaflet, 7, 62
PEM see Prescription event monitoring
Pharmaceutical development see Drug development
Pharmaceutical industry
    careers, 99–105
    interface with medical profession, 57–65
    obligations of, 44–45
    reporting to, 85–87
    response to adverse drug reactions, 64–65
    role in surveillance, 9–10, 67–75
Pharmacoepidemiology, 31, 120
Pharmacokinetics, 17, 49, 120
    half life, 18
    steady state, 49
Pharmacovigilance, 93
Phase I see Clinical Trials, phase I
Phase II see Clinical trials, phase II
Phase III see Clinical trials, phase III
Phase IV see Clinical trials, phase IV

PMS see Post-marketing surveillance
Post-marketing surveillance, 3, 4, 27–36, 120
    studies, 32–33, 103
PPA see Prescription Pricing Authority
Prescribing Analysis and Costs, 40
Prescribing information see Data sheet
Prescription event monitoring, 33–34, 107, 120
Prescription Pricing Authority, 30, 34, 35
Private health plans, 36
Product liability see Liability
Product licence application, 1, 25, 90, 101, 106
    appeal, 93
    granting, 92
    refusal, 93
Prophylaxis, 28
Protocol, 20, 22, 23
Published reports see Case reports

Randomization, 29
Rechallenge, 49, 50–51, 58, 70, 121
Record linkage, 35, 107, 121
Regional ADR centres, 78, 106
Regulatory authorities, 89–97
    careers, 106
    reporting to, 77–85
    reports from, 69
    requirements, 6
Regulatory report, 23, 104
    domestic, 96
    foreign, 94, 96
Report forms see Adverse event forms; Regulatory reports
Reporting
    adverse drug reactions, 77–78
        by pharmacists, 82
        established drugs, 82
        new drugs, 78–82
    barriers to, 59–60
    ethical dilemmas, 59
    fraudulent, 61
    non-medically qualified persons, 63
    payment for, 64
    rates, 42
    reasons for, 58
    see also Pharmaceutical industry; Regulatory authorities
Risk-factors, 30, 40, 44
    profiles, 27
    subgroups at particular risk, 73

Safety, Efficacy and Adverse Reaction Subcommittee, 95, 121

Scottish Hospital Morbidity Returns,
35
SEAR *see* Safety, Efficacy and Adverse
Reaction Subcommittee
Security, 61
SEDBASE, 111
Serious reactions
examples of, 80–81
pharmaceutical company definition,
85
regulatory definition, 82
suspected, 43
Side-effects, 1, 121
common, 8
Signal generation, 10
see also Hypothesis generation
Spontaneous reports
comparison with different drugs, 41–
42
Spontaneous reporting, 4, 37–45, 121
factors influencing, 42–43
role, 38–42
source, 43
Statistics, 22–23
Stratification, 31
Strict liability *see* Liability

Teratogenicity, 114
see also Toxicological evaluation,
teratogenicity
Thalidomide, 37, 89
Time to onset, 49–50, 60, 70

Toxicity
organ specific toxicity, 16
toxicological evaluation, 14–16, 92
acute, 14–15
Ames test, 16
carcinogenicity, 14, 15
fertility, 14, 15
LD_{50}, 15
multiple dose, 15
teratogenicity, 14, 15, 92, 115
see also Animal toxicity
Type A *see* Adverse drug reactions, type
A
Type B *see* Adverse drug reactions, type
B

Under-reporting, 38

Vaccines
adverse reactions to, 84
Veterans association, 36
Voluntary reporting *see* Spontaneous
reporting

WHO *see* World Health Organization
Withdrawal from market, 39
World Health Organization, 95, 121

Yellow Card, 34, 78–84, 121
information on, 84–85
number of reports, 78